LIFE, DEATH, AND DECISIONS

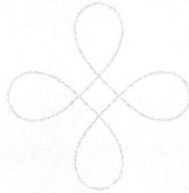

Puxiao Cen, MD, FACC

THIS BOOK IS DEDICATED TO

MY LATE FATHER

DOCTOR AND PROFESSOR ZEBO CEN

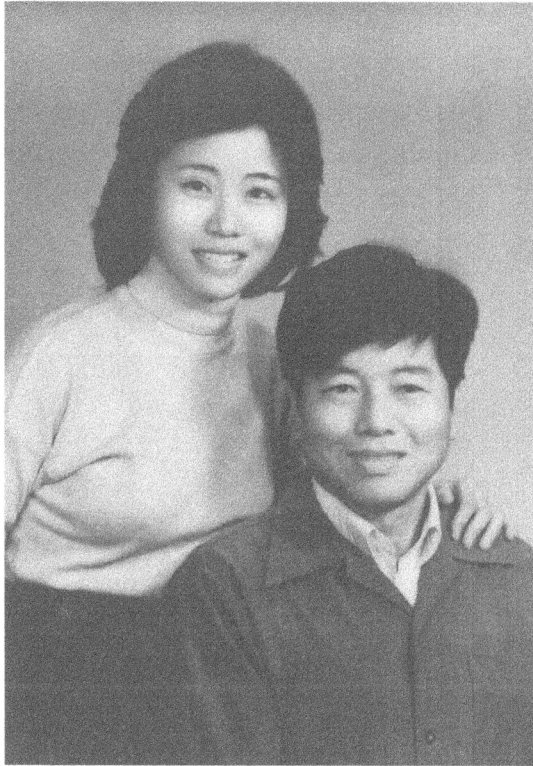

Doctor Puxiao Cen and her late father

FOREWORD

Nanette K. Wenger

MD, MACC, MACP, FAHA

Professor of Medicine (Cardiology)
Emory University School of Medicine Consultant
Emory Heart and Vascular Center Founding Consultant
Emory Women's Heart Center Atlanta, GA

Multiple academic presentations have reviewed the pillars of bioethics in healthcare: beneficience, non-maleficence, autonomy, confidentiality, and justice. But how are these concepts incorporated and implemented in daily clinical practice? How are these manifest in physician-patient interactions? The contemporary practice of U.S. medicine, the professionalism of medicine, involves social contracts between providers of healthcare, their patients, the community, and the insurers—based on these ethical principles of beneficience, non-maleficence, autonomy, and justice, with social justice posing special challenges. In our increasingly diverse society, cultural sensitivity becomes an important interface with these ethical issues. Economic inequality challenges social justice and compounds healthcare inequalities, yet physicians and their patients interact within these constraints in daily healthcare encounters.

In "Life, Death, and Decisions" Dr. Puxiao Cen displays the unique approach of Case Studies, followed by relevant ethical issues, and poses questions based on the discussion topics, e.g., - end-of-life care, undocumented immigrants, interface of medicine and the law, access to healthcare, etc. Justice and equity in healthcare pose challenges to the appropriate implementation of healthcare policy and allocation of healthcare resources, particularly to vulnerable populations.

In both the clinical and the research arenas, the physician-patient interface provides the opportunity for the physician to inform the patient about his or her disease and to outline the preferred diagnostic and therapeutic approaches—including, importantly, consideration of patient preferences. However, as displayed in Aristotle's Rhetoric, this essentially involves persuasion, i.e., the art of persuasion becomes important because it allows the truth to win over lies. The description by Aristotle of the 3 methods of persuasion has high relevance for clinical practice. First of the 3 methods is persuasion by character or credibility, i.e., people who appear trustworthy—with the trustworthy person typified as having good sense, good moral character, and goodwill. This involves being a competent and credible physician in the topic under discussion, providing the patient with the relevant facts, explaining the potential consequences of the relative choices, and having the best interests of the patient at heart. That this is done in a calm and caring manner, importantly identifying the physician's concern for patient preferences and desired outcomes of the healthcare encounter, transfers to the clinical setting what Aristotle promulgated in terms of statesmanship and community values. This persuasion by character Aristotle defines as ethos. The ethos, i.e., the credibility or ethical appeal, is as relevant today as it was in the 4th century BC; although Aristotle was addressing decision-making as a policy situation in the public arena, the effort to insure the best outcomes applies equally to the physician-patient interactions.

The second approach to persuasion per Aristotle is persuasion by emotion, or pathos. Here he emphasizes calm as contrasted with anger, friendship as contrasted with hatred, confidence as contrasted with fear and kindness as contrasted with being unkind. The optimal persuader is defined by Aristotle as using the emotions appropriately; persuasion involves an argument that is sound and builds on logic that is easy to follow. Aristotle concludes that this rhetoric is important because it helps the truth prevail, citing that because some people cannot be convinced by facts alone it is important to know how to persuade them. He advocates that knowing how to leverage character, emotion, and logic can help bring the desired changes. Effective physician rhetoric thus involves knowing the audience (your patient), knowing the topic (the clinical problem), and choosing the appropriate language. Emotions are powerful motivators, so that the optimal approach is not solely fact and discussion and emotion, but a combination of all three.

Given the initial emphasis on the personal character of the speaker (ethos) and the frame of mind of the patient or recipient (pathos), the third approach relates to the proof generated by the presentation itself (logos). Ethos is essentially an appeal to the ethics, convincing the recipient of the credibility of the speaker. Pathos, an appeal to the emotion, creates a response to a personal direction. Logos, the appeal to logic, is the way one uses facts and figures.

Translated from the Aristotelian sphere into the clinical encounter, it requires that ethical principles be used in this approach to physician-patient shared decision-making, with the goal of informing, persuading and motivating the patient.

Highly relevant to the contemporary political, social, and judicial rhetoric is social justice and equity in healthcare for vulnerable populations, specifically as addressed by the Patient Protection and Affordable Care Act of 2010 (ACA). Community health centers in both rural and urban settings were federally funded, with some regional and local support. Patients were not excluded by their lack of ability to pay and were offered primary medical, dental, behavioral, and social services in medically underserved areas. Also within the ACA is the National Health Services Corps of primary care physicians who provide basic medical services to vulnerable Americans in underserved areas. Expanding the access to medical care both in underserved urban and rural communities, with these safety net systems, provides for the care of individual patients and enhances the health status of the target populations. The desired impact is social justice and healthcare equity for vulnerable populations.

Nowhere are ethical principles more integral to the discussions than in medical research involving human subjects where important issues of both individual protections and community protections are raised. Informed consent involving genetic research demands precise ethical attention to short- and long-term consequences. In a chapter addressing the advances in therapeutic cloning, the potential to achieve organ transplantation without a donor and without the need for immunosuppressive therapy, benefit is balanced against potential risks. These risks and benefits have been debated in medical, political, and legal arenas, with the advances in technology at the frontier of improving outcomes.

The Case Studies at the end of the book are challenging and poignant. They define the intersection of medical practice and the law, in some instances where laws likely should have been superceded by contemporary knowledge. These cases are not intended to provide answers but rather to foster discussion—discussion of where social change may be needed, where political change may be needed, and/or where legal change may be requisite. Optimal forums include grand rounds, journal clubs, medical staff meetings, IRB meetings, professional society congresses, and public-professional convocations. The emphasis for all discussions is that the patients' rights and protections should be foremost, rather than a focus predominantly on liability.

I thoroughly enjoyed reading (and studying) this monograph and enthusiastically recommend it to my colleagues.

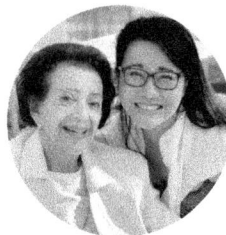

Dr. Nanette K. Wenger and Dr. Puxiao Cen

ABOUT THE AUTHOR

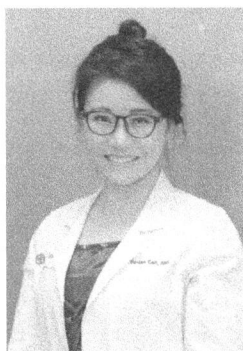

Dr. Puxiao Cen is an invasive cardiologist, board-certified in internal medicine, cardiovascular disease, advanced heart failure and transplant cardiology, nuclear cardiology, and adult echocardiography. She has been a Fellow of the American College of Cardiology since 2003 and has been caring for the people of the Orlando, FL area for 25 years. Puxiao is also a physician member of the Medical Ethics Committee for the area health system and Assistant Professor at the University of Central Florida, College of Medicine. Puxiao doesn't just absorb all that the world has to offer and keep that learning and knowledge locked away inside her. Dr. Cen considers it her mission to process and refine the knowledge she has gained from her experiences and distill it down to the salient points so she can recommunicate that knowledge in a manner that can benefit everyone. That philosophy was the motivation behind writing *Life,*

Death, and Decisions. Dr. Cen wants to help impart some of the lessons she has learned as a medical ethicist in a major health system to the general public. By doing so, she hopes that the healthcare professional, patients, their families, and the communities in which they live can better navigate the modern world of healthcare. Even though this book is being published during the middle of the COVID-19 pandemic, Puxiao actually completed the book in late 2018, so there are no case studies or references to COVID19 in the book. However, the basic principles discussed in the book are foundational to understanding medical ethics and can be applied to patient care and research ethics during the pandemic.

CONTENTS

Chapter 1

Cultural Context—Lost in Translation

Often in healthcare ethics we examine values through the lenses of philosophy and religion. We should also incorporate other perspectives or filters to determine how meaning is made and who can/should/does control how that is done. We can employ anthropology, globalization, US health care, power issues and autonomy as backdrops to consider that which is not overt in many bioethics discussions.

Discussion Topics

How is the context of the body both an internal and an external feature in how a life is lived?

The story of Caitlyn Jenner has brought the topic of how a life is lived to the forefront of people's minds. Caitlyn saw herself as a man and an Olympic athlete when she was Bruce Jenner and society perceived her as such. But, at some point Bruce's internal conception of who he was changed, and he knew that he was a woman. Once he came to terms with that idea, he took steps to transform his external appearance to match his internal perception of himself. Society then had to adjust the way it collectively perceived and received Caitlyn Jenner. This change of body context was generated from within Bruce and required active external changes to his body to cause society to adjust its perception of who Bruce/Caitlyn actually is.

Interestingly, Sharon Kaufman, in her paper about "death with dignity," turned the topic of changing appearance around in her discussion about Mrs. Sato and Mrs. Peterson.[01] Both Mrs. Sato and Mrs. Peterson did not change their bodies and their physical presence in the world from an act of volition, but rather had the changes forced upon them by nature. Unlike patients who are able to adjust their internal, mental conception of self in response to their disease, Mrs. Sato and Mrs. Peterson could not make any internal, mental changes to their reality. Rather, Sato and Peterson had their reality defined by those around them. This is important because Kaufman is able to show how two patients

01 Kaufman, S. R. (2000). In the shadow of "death with dignity": Medicine and cultural quandaries of the vegetative state. *American Anthropologist, 102*(1), 69-83.

with very similar presentations live strikingly different lives and have different futures based on how their body is defined within the context created by those around them.

The idea that internal and external forces are constantly at play defining a patient is an important consideration for healthcare providers. We can adjust how we approach patient care based on how the context is changing.

The Premier Exhibitions' website for "Bodies... the Exhibition" presents images and information for "over 200 actual human bodies and specimens meticulously dissected and respectfully displayed, offering an unprecedented and wholly unique view into the amazing body." The exhibit provides an opportunity for discussion about the ethics of the source of the bodies as well as the content of the display.

After exploring the "Bodies...the Exhibition" website, there were three things that stood out to me: 1) the origin of the bodies; 2) the intent of the exhibit; and 3) the content of the exhibit. There has been controversy over the origin of the bodies presented in the "Bodies" exhibit. The website only indicates in the disclaimer that the company managing the exhibit "cannot independently verify that [the human remains] do not belong to persons executed while incarcerated in Chinese prisons."[01] In a 2008 interview for the television program 20/20, a Chinese medical technician named Deqiang Sun claimed to have "illegally acquired the bodies of executed prisoners to be dissected and injected with plastic by a Chinese company that prepares bodies for public display."[02] Given

01 Premier Exhibitions, Inc. (2014). Retrieved from http://www.premierexhibitions.com/exhibitions/4/4/bodies-exhibition/bodies-exhibition-disclaimer

02 Schwartz, R. (2010, December 8). The "Body Show" battles: Rival exhibitors square off in court. Retrieved from http://abcnews.go.com/Blotter/body-show-battles-rival-exhibitors-square-off-court/story?id=12348566

China's long history of human rights violations, one might tend to agree with the individuals who claim that the bodies do indeed include the remains of people tortured and killed while prisoners in China.

The intent and presentation of the exhibit were areas that seem slightly incongruous on the website showing images from the exhibit. The website seems to push the image of an educational exhibition of the human body for school-aged children, but the actual presentation seems to be more like a circus sideshow intent on titillation and shock. There are certain aspects of the exhibit, such as the bodies arranged in sexual positions, that even I, as a physician, would not have wanted my son to see as a young child.

Some of the content of the exhibition seems to push the boundaries of that which is ethical. Much of the exhibition comes across as exploitative of the people who may have unwilling donated their bodies. This is particularly true of the fetuses that are displayed in jars. Certainly, the fetuses could not give permission and one might guess that permission may not have been sought from the parents of the fetuses given the uncertainty about the provenance of the adult bodies.

As a whole, "Bodies...the Exhibition" places the human body in a context that makes one wonder if one is participating in violating the autonomy of the people whose bodies are on display.

Of Arthur Frank's four body types, which one speaks most clearly to you and why?

Arthur Frank's *The Wounded Storyteller* attempts to explain why suffering needs stories, stories of our own suffering and of other people's. The book is not only about the types of stories of suffering that we tell and how to recognize the purposes of these stories, but also how to listen to stories and the storyteller. Frank identifies four body types that exist in illness narratives: the disciplined body, mirroring body, dominating body, and communicative body. None of these body types can exist in singularity, but all play a greater or lesser role from time to time in one way or another. These bodies are attitudes towards the illness and the ordeals the ill body faces. The disciplined body prioritizes the demands of getting well over other desires. The mirroring body finds identity by modeling other bodies. Its desire is to be as healthy as the bodies shown in advertisements. The dominating body is one that attempts to control others because his/her own body is out of control. The communicative body is the idealized type for an illness narrative because it uses communion and communication of stories to define itself in relation to others.

When I was younger, I probably was more strongly aligned with the disciplined body type. Discipline is a stereotype of Chinese born and raised in mainland China, but it happens to be true. Whether I was focused on academics or training for the city swim team, my life revolved around controlling myself and my environment to the best of my ability. But, as Frank states, "no actual body fits [the disciplined, mirroring, and dominating body type] specifications, at least for long, but these specifications... [help one understand] how bodies exist at different moments of their being."[03] I learned how true this was when I was diagnosed with stage 2 ovarian cancer in 2007. As hard as I tried to control everything about my treatment and my body, I was forced to stand by and watch as the surgical treatment stole my ovaries and my uterus. Then the chemotherapy sapped my strength, sickened me, and made my hair fall out. Eventually, I had to acknowledge that control was just an illusion and suddenly I shifted away from being a disciplined body to bouncing among the other body types depending on the day, how I felt, and a thou-

---

03 Frank, A. (1995). *The wounded storyteller: Body, illness, and ethics*. Chicago, IL: University of Chicago Press.

sand other factors. Even after my recovery and being cancer-free I still need to accept that there are some lingering reminders that I cannot hope to control everything in my life or my body. I have lingering neuropathy in my hands from the chemotherapy and I am not longer able to perform cardiac catheterization which was something I loved about being a cardiologist. I absolutely agree that by embracing the disease and the sequelae, one can come to terms with one's new reality.

What do the ideas of context introduce into the interpretive structure of bioethics?

Arthur Kleinman's "constrained relativism" reminds me of Shirley Jackson's story, *The Lottery*, about a society where a lottery is used to select a human sacrifice to ensure the community's continued well-being. Relativism, when taken to extremes, can be deemed unethical, but when applied to situations in a "constrained", limited way can prove to provide useful context when addressing a patient's healthcare needs. When applied at an appropriate level, taking into account a patient's cultural background and the context of her life can prove beneficial to gaining a patient's respect and trust. This in turn would help to drive patient engagement and ownership in her healthcare.

This type of engagement can be important when attempting to implement a new healthcare program in an ethnic minority community. Over time, there have been missteps when dealing with minority communities such as during the Tuskegee Syphilis Study or the Havasupai Tribe's lawsuit against Arizona State University for inappropriate use of medical samples for genetic testing. Once trust is lost in the medical establishment by a minority group, it is hard to regain that trust. However, while understanding and giving consideration to an individual's life context is useful, it is not the only factor to consider when treating a patient. So, context adds to the application of bioethics to healthcare provision, but it is only one aspect to consider out of many factors impacting medical ethics.

How does one's personal/communal context shape one's view of the world, however one might define that view?

The response of different ethnic groups to the use of genetic testing provides unexpected insight into how one's communal identity influences one's worldview. Resistance and skepticism towards genetic testing has been seen across several different cultural and social groups. One example is the situation experienced by the Havasupai Indian Tribe who agreed to submit blood samples to researchers at Arizona State University to search for a link to diabetes. Unfortunately, the medical team decided to use the Havasupai samples for other research including schizophrenia, migration patterns and inbreeding which violated the basic rule of human based research ethics. The use of genetic information to analyze migration patterns and thereby speculate at the accuracy of the tribe's origin may create significant conflict with and among the members of the tribe. If the tribe's identity is tied to the how their ancestors came to exist, and that story is proven false, then the entire basis for the tribe's cultural beliefs come into question. In order to protect their cultural identity and their worldview, the Havasupai Tribe refused to allow the genetic testing to be communicated and published.

This type of resistance to genetic testing also exists among the African American community. As ethicists Beeson and Doksum argue "personal resistance to genetic testing explicitly is linked to the larger social implications of such practices."[04] The main crux of the distrust that dominated

---

04 Beeson, D., & Doksum, T. (2001). Family values and resistance to genetic testing. In B. Hoffmaster (Ed.), *Bioethics in social context* (pp. 153-179). Philadelphia: Temple University Press.

an African American mother's viewpoint was the knowledge, in her mind, that the genetic testing will be used to discriminate against people. As she put it, "the facts are, have been, and will be that there will be discrimination. There will be unfair treatment of a lot of people as this becomes the rule of thumb or the order of the day, when it shouldn't be like that."[05]

People from a different social and cultural context have a different response to genetic testing simply because of having a different worldview due to living in a different social and cultural context. However, even a group of people who might be considered to have a universal worldview, such as the gay community, might have a difference of opinion. For instance, the gay community is divided about whether finding genetic links to homosexuality is good or not.[06] Those in the gay community who advocate genetic testing to find a gay gene believe that "linking homosexuality to genes shows that homosexual orientation is "natural" and implies that gays should not be blamed, stigmatized, or discriminated against for an orientation that arises from their genetic makeup."[07] Those concerned about genetic testing for homosexuality fear that it would lead to "remedicalization" of homosexuality with the consequent fetal testing and possible abortions and eugenics.[08] One might readily agree that the cultural context provided by one's tribe, community, or social group will impact and influence the worldviews of members of those groups.

---

05 Beeson, D., & Doksum, T. (2001). Family values and resistance to genetic testing. In B. Hoffmaster (Ed.), *Bioethics in social context* (pp. 153-179). Philadelphia: Temple University Press.

06 Ibid.

07 Conrad, P. (2001). Media images, genetics, and culture: Potential impacts of reporting scientific findings on bioethics. In B. Hoffmaster (Ed.), *Bioethics and social context* (pp. 90-111). Philadelphia: Temple University Press.

08 Ibid.

The possibility of abortions and eugenics is certainly alarming for many. Given the increased tolerance for gay persons in today's society, is there some merit to working at the level of social justice in the present in anticipation of new biotechnological capacities in the future?

There is an absolute necessity to anticipate the implication of future biotechnological advances and craft policy beforehand to help manage those advances. Genetics is one of the most controversial areas that we should address in the near term. The implications of advances in genetic testing and genetic engineering can be devastating to individuals and society as a whole. Besides the possibility for the "gay gene" being used to persecute, ostracize, and eradicate homosexuals, we need to consider the fact that genetic engineering can lead to people being discriminated against because they are predisposed to certain medical conditions. Insurance companies may be inclined to increase premiums, copayments, out of pocket requirements and limit maximum lifetime benefits based on genetic testing. Employers may also look for reasons not to hire people or terminate existing employees based on the potential cost to insure those individuals or the possibility of future disability claims or lost time from work due to genetic predispositions.

Policy also needs to be implemented to address the future potential for cloning of individuals for ethically questionable acts such as creating babies that are a perfect genetic match to an individual just to harvest tissues and organs for transplantation. If we do not engage in discussion and debate prior to biotech advances having real-world applications, we will have an insurmountable task ahead of us trying to scramble and implement last minute laws and policies.

When the discussion turns to genomics and mapping the human genome, the primary concerns seem to gravitate toward the fear of eugenics, cloning, and other discriminatory applications of the information derived from genetic testing. According to the genetic research team of McEwen et al., "the shift that is occurring in the field of genomics from an emphasis on basic research ... toward an emphasis on research with identified human participants and immediate clinical applications ... raises an expanded array of ethical issues, which the Ethical, Legal, and Social Implications (ELSI) Program is increasingly being called upon to address."[09] There seems to be readily evident concerns of the ELSI projects that are being addressed because of awareness. The light shone on problems or potential problems simply by increasing awareness and educating people seems to be invaluable in fomenting change or obviating the problem in the first place.

However, when ELSI is viewed through the filter of normativity of ethics research, the focus changed slightly for me and shifted to concerns about who was doing the research and what views/opinions the investigators represent. Catherine Myser, in particular, seems to set a pessimistic tone for the interpretation of ELSI with her essay on normativity of whiteness in bioethics.[10] Myser's opinion provides food for thought about considering different socio-cultural contexts when evaluating bioethics principles in research and the development of "bioethics theories, knowledge, methods, and policies."[11] Myser is a little bleak in her view when compared to the other extant literature on bioethics, all of which indicate that future bioethics theories, method, knowledge, and policies will be inclusive and consider the socio-cultural context of individuals im-

---

09 McEwen, J., Boyer, J., Sun, K., Rothenberg, K., Lockhart, N. & Guyer, M. (2014). The ethical, legal, and social implications program of the national human genome research institute: Reflections on an ongoing experiment. *The Annual Review of Genomics and Human Genetics.* 15:481–505 doi: 10.1146/annurev-genom-090413-025327

10 Myser, C. (2003). Differences from somewhere: The normativity of whiteness in bioethics in the United States. *American Journal of Bioethics, 3*(2), 1-11.

11 Ibid.

pacted by medical research and practice. I guess I am more hopeful that people actually learn from history and truly intend to do good to others.

Taking that into account, the ELSI projects are confronted by the problem of ensuring that the investigators will be objective, intellectually independent, and morally honest. One of the main barriers to maintaining the integrity of the system is the fact that the ELSI program is housed within the same structure that supports the science being researched. If the ELSI projects can be insulated from any questions of integrity and maintain some indication of inculcating socio-cultural context into bioethical theory development, then ELSI may be able to facilitate the conduct of genomic science in an ethically, legally, and socially responsible way.

Some people might question the down-the-road implications of the use of the research data. To take the thought process a step further, not only must we worry about who is using the data and for what purpose, but we must also worry about who may be adversely impacted by the data. In addition to the potential for an Orwell-meets-Maslow type of genetic purification in the future, we might also want to consider the unfortunate potential for targeting and culling of certain ethnic or social groups based on genetic profiling.

Genetic testing is not only a biomedical procedure, but also a way of creating social categories. As a basic principle, we believe that people should be evaluated based on their individual merits and abilities, and not based on stereotypes and predictions about their future performance or health status. Usually, genetic testing can only point to probabilities or potentialities and not necessarily absolute certainties. We believe that individuals should not be judged based on stereotypes and assumptions about what people in their class or status are like. Genetic data can indeed be misused and abused to target certain groups of people which makes transparency of who is doing what and why they are doing it all the more crucial in the ELSI Programs.

My main point is that it is difficult to see the socio-cultural background and ideology of the people conducting the ELSI research project and studies. By comparing Myser's focus on the "whiteness" that she suggests predominates biomedical research with the ELSI's lack of transparency, one can see the implication of this lack of transparency in that certain ethnic or social groups might be targeted for discrimination.

Medical Anthropological Research and Global Views on Stigma

Arthur Kleinman's presentation, "Medical Anthropology and Mental Health: Five Questions for the Future Society for Medial Anthropology" at Yale University in September 2009, posed one question in particular that struck a chord with me. The question that interested me was Kleinman's query that "if ... ground zero for patients with psychosis globally is moral death and social exclusion, what is the implication for medical anthropological research of going beyond stigma to redefine what is at stake in the most severe psychiatric conditions in cultural terms?".[12] Kleinman, a psychiatrist and professor of medical anthropology and cross-cultural psychiatry, has spoken about this several times over the years and he has consistently opined that "understanding the unique social and cultural processes that create stigma in the lived worlds of the stigmatised should be the first focus of our efforts to combat stigma."[13] I agree with Kleinman's assessment that gaining an understanding of the root cause and contributing factors behind stigmatization within a

---

12 Kleinman, A. (2009, September). *Medical Anthropology and Mental Health: Five Questions for the Future Society for Medial Anthropology.* Paper presented at Society of Medical Anthropology Meeting, Yale University.

13 Kleinman, A. & Hall-Clifford, R. (2009). Stigma: A social, cultural and moral process. *Journal of Epidemiology and Community Health.* 63:418–419. doi:10.1136/jech.2008.084277

society is vital to reversing the effects of stigma.

Because a great deal of Kleinman's research has been performed in China and Taiwan, I feel a special interest in his theories. Kleinman's discussion of people in China who suffer from schizophrenia, HIV/ AIDS, leprosy, or epilepsy often facing social marginalization because of their illnesses was quite accurate from my experience. Chinese society can be unforgiving of those who are outside the physical or mental standard for "normal." From Kleinman's experience, people with stigmas "lose their moral face" and "are not considered human."[14] In China, the concept of "face" has been in existence for centuries and would be extremely hard to overcome. Anything that causes a person to "lose face" is to be avoided and not discussed. Kleinman believes that the solution to the problems of stigmatization will come from unintentional cultural changes which have been happening over the past couple of decades that eventually strip mental illnesses of stigma.

I agree with Kleinman's opinion that using both quantitative and qualitative research efforts can contribute to a scientific study of stigma and that epidemiology can inform ethnographic research on the causes, course and potential solutions for stigma. By utilizing this type of multidisciplinary approach to stigma, academic and medical research and public policy can come together to create anti-stigma interventions that have real and measurable outcomes.

Structural Violence and Context-dependent Respect for Autonomy

At times I wonder if we, as a species, are ever going to be able to get beyond the "us *vs.* them" mentality that leads to structural violence. I am reminded of Jane Elliott's "Blue eyes–Brown eyes" exercise that she did

---

14 Ibid.

with her elementary school class the day after Martin Luther King, Jr. was shot on April 4, 1968. The exercise was filmed in 1970 with her third-grade class and became the educational film "Eye of the Storm." Elliott's exercise was basically dividing the class into two groups by eye color, blue-eyed children in one group and brown-eyed children in the other group.

On that first day of the exercise, Elliott gave the blue-eyed children and extra privileges and made them sit at the front of the class. The brown-eyed children had to sit in the back of the class and were often criticized. The change in the children's behavior was startling. The "superior" children became arrogant, bossy, and otherwise unpleasant to their "inferior" classmates. Their grades on simple tests were better, and they completed mathematical and reading tasks that had seemed outside their ability before. The "inferior" classmates became timid and subservient children who scored more poorly on tests, and even during recess isolated themselves, including those who had previously been dominant in the class. These children's academic performance suffered, even with tasks that had been simple before.

The next Monday, Elliott reversed the exercise, making the brown-eyed children superior. While the brown-eyed children did taunt the blue-eyed children in ways similar to what had occurred the previous day, Elliott reports it was much less intense. This exercise is often used as an example of how prejudice can form and the impact that prejudice (us *vs.* them) can have on minority sectors of society. While, some academic research into Elliott's exercise shows moderate results in reducing long-term prejudice, there is still the question of whether the possible psychological harm outweighs the potential benefits. Even though there is some conjecture as to whether the exercise was unethical and psychologically/emotionally damaging, the take home message is that simply by labels and the support of authority figures, one group within society can oppress another group and fail to acknowledge the wants and needs of the minority group. This superiority vs. inferiority dynamic can play a very damaging role in the implementation of structural violence that can impact the provision of healthcare.

Chinese Society and Structural Violence

The current notion of personhood in Chinese society is firmly rooted in thousands of years of culture. While there are a few rumblings among people for social change, especially in humanitarian terms, change will be difficult to undertake. The current changes that the world has witnessed China experience over the last several years has been a calculated economic decision after witnessing the collapse of the USSR and the rest of the Soviet Bloc. The relative economic strength of China is really isolated to the major cities and the political figures in the Communist Party and those with political influence. The rural areas outside the major cities lack civil engineering infrastructure and financial stability which includes poor access to healthcare services.

China has historically been ruled by an absolute dictator, whether he was called Emperor or Chairman the effect has been the same, and the populace has become accustomed to living that way. This even led to the atrocities of the Cultural Revolution where families were torn apart and children reported parents for "subversive" behavior. Many people were thrown into prison or executed because they did not follow the edicts of the Party...and that was less than 50 years ago.

There will not be a Martin Luther King, Jr. or Abraham Lincoln in China. Chinese society is not structured like America. My father was a brilliant orthopedic surgeon in China and because of his expertise was able to get away with never joining the Communist Party. Not long after my younger sister was born, the one child policy was implemented. Should my mother have gotten pregnant a year later, she would have been forced to have an abortion. This is not the type of society where one can see an avenue to changing the society's view of the mental ill. The stigma will remain until the government falls and the populace has a chance to be exposed to different ideas and cultural concepts without censorship or fear. Just like we must consider context when thinking about medical care, we must think about context when thinking about social/structural change. You can make a recommendation about what road China should take, but that is the same as a doctor telling a patient what treatment is best for them. The patient might not agree based on his or her cultural context.

Technology has become the major form of "caregiving" in the biomedical project—Good, Bad, or Meh?

My first inclination was to write about the love affair that the healthcare system has with the EMR and the way everyone is chasing that unicorn even though there is no agreed upon platform or universal standard for the industry. Then I thought I should write about the growth of defensive medicine as a prophylactic against malpractice charges to show conscientious medical practice. I have certainly seen this increase almost exponentially over my last 20 years of medical practice. But these are fairly obvious targets for discussion.

One area that caught me off guard was the interplay between fertility treatments and technology. That had not occurred to me to be an area where technology was feeding into the growth of medical use and expense beyond what was necessary or useful for the good of society. Margarete Sandelowski's article about the never-enough quality of conceptive technology is of interest because of her theories about the effect of society forces and pressures on the changing role of technology in fertility and, consequently, the disproportionate growth of fertility treatments in light of the low success rates. Even though the success rate of IVF is higher than the outdated rate quoted by Sandelowski, this points to the way society focuses on the "need" to achieve almost any biomedical outcome that can, or maybe "should," be reached through the investment in, and the application of, technology.

From a personal point of view, my husband and I tried to have a second child later in life. So, after a few years of trying and failing to become pregnant, we decided to go to a fertility doctor. I am not so sure that we would have made the same decision if we were without the financial wherewithal to cover the expense with negligible impact to our lives. This fact reminds me of Sandelowski's conjecture that "conceptive technology requires human beings to determine and achieve its purposes, but it also has an inherent quality of never being enough."[15] We were prepared to exhaust every possible technological advancement to become pregnant. We were stopped midstream because part of the diagnostic process was a hysteroscopy and hysterosalpingogram which showed what was thought to be an ovarian cyst, but turned out to be ovarian cancer. Even during the discussion about surgical removal of the ovaries, we considered options to harvest eggs for later fertilization and implantation. The persistence in treatment for infertility is quite real and deceptive. It creeps into your rational brain and changes the decision-making landscape in such a way that leads to the "confusion of the good with the sufficient."[16]

Implications of technology as the major form of "caregiving" in the world of biomedical healthcare

Some may consider the impact of healthcare technology on the human

---

15 Sandelowski, M. (1991). Compelled to try: The never-enough quality of conceptive technology. *Medical Anthropology Quarterly, 5*(1), 29-47.

16 Sandelowski, M. (1991). Compelled to try: The never-enough quality of conceptive technology. *Medical Anthropology Quarterly, 5*(1), 29-47.

psyche to create a condition in which people would use technology to realize a desire to live in the world, yet remain untouched by the world. Lawler, in his paper "Caregiving and the American Individual," addressed this concept of "[l]ives moved by a veneration of independence threaten to leave us unprepared for depending and being depended upon."[17] Lawler seems to lay the price of our ability to provide for basic human needs at the feet of technological advancement. Maybe one can say that the focus on extraordinary measures, or pushing the boundaries of what is medically possible, makes ordinary biomedical needs seem too prosaic to address as more than an afterthought.[18] Have we as a species, especially in America, become too entranced with technology to the exclusion of the social aspects of caregiving?

Humans seem to have a great desire to fight against the Second Law of Thermodynamics. Entropy dominates the world in which we live and our intolerance of entropy leads us to constantly seek ways to halt the ceaseless march of time. We fight our enemy Entropy in our external environment (repainting our houses, manicuring our landscapes, replacing our vehicles, etc.) and our internal environment (knee replacement surgery, cardiac stent placement, HGH injections, etc.). Technology has been our best (or maybe easiest to use) weapon in the war we wage against entropy, time, and disease. Interestingly, from my experience as a cardiologist, patients are more likely to eschew low tech interventions such as diet and exercise in favor of technological advances such as medications and surgical interventions to address healthcare concerns. This is interesting to me because industrialized nations with longer than expected average life expectancies, such as the Okinawans, point to diet and lifestyle as

---

17 Lawler, P. A. (2004). *Caregiving and the American individual*. Publication of The President's Council on Bioethics.

18   Ibid.

the reason for the extended lifespan, not medical interventions. In fact, the US spends far more on healthcare than any other country, yet the life expectancy of the American population is actually shorter than in other countries that spend far less.[19] The hunger for easy solutions (technology) to a difficult problem (human entropy) seems to point to a cultural shift within the US as the wellspring of technology is simply the tool of choice. The implications are frightening because one must wonder how far we are going to travel down this technological road in pursuit of longer life at the expense of our collective, communal humanity.

Impact of technology on healthcare decision-making

The negative impacts of technology through financial strain and societal expectation fit quite well with the idea that physicians have increasingly engaged in what has come to be called "defensive medicine." We can look at defensive medicine as the practice of physicians ordering tests and procedures, making referrals or taking other treatment steps with the main impetus being to help protect themselves from liability rather than to benefit their patients' care. A 2013 study published in Health Affairs found that physicians reporting a high level of malpractice concern were most likely to engage in practices that would be considered defensive (for example, more aggressive diagnostic testing) when diagnosing patients with new complaints of chest pain, headache, or lower back pain.[20] From discussions I have had with other physicians, there is a fear of litigation because physicians tend to think that patients, and a jury of their peers, will always think that one more test could have been done or a higher

---

19 Ibid.

20 Packer-Tursman, J. (2015). The defensive medicine balancing act. *Medical Economics*. Retrieved from http://infoweb.newsbank.com.cuhsl.creighton.edu/resources/doc/nb/news/15376756B9C19560?p=AWNB

tech intervention could have been performed. Vikas Saini, MD, president of the Lown Institute, sees "the problem of unnecessary care and use as a deep cultural problem, I can sum it up as more is not always better, but that is the cultural bias."[21] This takes on a slightly different hue when viewed through the context lens of a demanding profession. As Saini puts it, "There's a lot of borderline. There's a lot of uncertainty, guessing. It is not purely defensive. There's also profound concern for your patient and concern for your reputation all wrapped together."[22] Practicing medicine with fear of unreasonable patient and public expectations of what could possibly be done given the vast amount of technology at our disposal is not beneficial for the physicians, the patients, the society, or the state of healthcare in America. A deeper, more deleterious issue is that modern medicine has become driven by technology and financial considerations, while we really need to be free to make decisions that are driven by patients' needs.

Impact of emotions on bioethics as a reflector, sustainer, and perpetuator of power relations

When ethicists Anspach and Beeson discuss emotions in medical and moral life, their statement, "Emotions reflect, sustain and perpetuate power relations" is not as absolute as the authors suggest when taken in the context of the medical environment.[23] A more nuanced consideration is required to fully evaluate the role of emotions in the dynamics of power relations. One must go beyond the initial relationship structure to

---

21 Ibid.

22 Ibid.

23 Anspach, R. R., & Beeson, D. (2001). Emotions in medical and moral life. In B. Hoffmaster (Ed.), *Bioethics in social context* (pp. 112-136). Philadelphia: Temple University Press.

ascertain whether emotion is a by-product of the situation or a driver for the situation. By default, a patient is going to be more emotionally invested in the patient-provider relationship than the medical provider because the relationship is all about "self" for the patient. In the case of the patient populations for Anspach and Beeson, we are talking about neonatal intensive care and genetic testing among pregnant women respectively. Both of the decision-making patient populations for these studies are in the position where the health and welfare of their child is in question and at risk. To say that the power relations between the patient and provider are being reflected, sustained, and perpetuated based on those scenarios is a misevaluation of the situation or at least a misattribution of the source of the power. Does the parents' emotional investment in the outcome of the situation make them inferior to the medical team? The structure would be the same sans emotion.

The impact on bioethics will depend on the individuals involved in the situation. As Robichaud notes, if "disharmonious disagreement over treatment options is being fueled by emotion, there is an obligation on the part of healthcare providers to directly address the role emotion is playing."[24] The impact would be the same as any other factor that might impact bioethics such as a lack of understanding a situation's cultural or ethnic context. One must remain cognizant of the impact of emotion on decision-making. As Cornell's psychology professor David Pizarro argues, "emotions reflect our pre-existing concerns, such as our moral beliefs and principles, making them less capricious than may appear. [E]motions can actually aid reasoning by acting as a centralizing agent, focusing our attention and our cognitive resources on the problem at hand."[25] By

---

24 Robichaud, A. L. (2003). Healing and feeling: The clinical ontology of emotion. *Bioethics, 17*(1), 59-68.

25 Pizarro, D. (2000). Nothing more than feelings? the role of emotions in moral judgment. *Journal for the Theory of Social Behaviour, 30*(4), 355-373.

focusing our attention, emotions can have a beneficial impact on moral decision-making and therefore the application of bioethics to medical practice.

Sustain and perpetuate—Semantics or pejorative intent?

I think the use of the words "sustain" and "perpetuate" led me to a more negative interpretation of their description of the nature of emotion. The underlying tone of Anspach and Beeson's article "Emotions in Medical and Moral Life" came across as if the authors had a preconceived theory and tried to provide anecdotal evidence to support that theory. I find it interesting that Anspach and Beeson consider that while "certain emotions, such as anger, are the exclusive prerogative of the powerful, emotionality is most likely to be attributed to dominated groups in society, such as women, children, and the lower classes."[26] That seems to presume that emotions are negative, or perceived to be a negative attribute, and used by those with power in a relationship to maintain or reinforce their superiority within the relationship. Moreover, anger in the medical field in not acceptable regardless of the perceived power relationship among the individuals involved. I would be more inclined to believe that a patient's emotions of pain or fear or sorrow would be taken as another factor that should be part of treating the whole patient. I tend to think that we have become more progressive in our approach to emotions in medical care than Anspach and Beeson give us credit for. In fact, I think we are closer to being in line with Pizarro's thought "that emotions should not be dismissed as irrelevant or harmful to moral evaluations, but

---

26 Anspach, R. R., & Beeson, D. (2001). Emotions in medical and moral life. In B. Hoffmaster (Ed.), *Bioethics in social context* (pp. 112-136). Philadelphia: Temple University Press.

that affect can actually aid moral deliberations."[27]

EQ—Recognize and know how you and others feel and react

The psychological theory of Emotional Intelligence has been a popular topic among business and leadership development folks. The theory suggests that people with a high degree of emotional intelligence know what they're feeling, what their emotions mean and how these emotions can affect other people. A leader would be expected to use this understanding of managing one's own emotions and those of the people around him or her to build a more cohesive, emotionally evolved team. If leaders have a solid understanding of how their emotions and actions affect the people around them, then emotions can be used to enhance the situation rather than detract from the situation. This means that the better a leader relates to and works with others, the more successful he or she will be. Therefore, in the biomedical environment, leaders who are cognizant of their emotions and those of their team (leaders who have a high degree of emotional intelligence) would theoretically be more responsive in bioethical decision-making.

The counter to this would be if a leader neglects to proactively address emotional issues with the medical team. In that case, the leader and the team would lose a wonderful opportunity to strengthen the shared purpose of the group. I think that shutting down the emotions of members of the medical team or of patients can cause the entire situation to come unraveled. Emotions play a very valuable role in sensing the gravity of ethical situations and responding appropriately.

---

27 Pizarro, D. (2000). Nothing more than feelings? the role of emotions in moral judgment. *Journal for the Theory of Social Behaviour, 30*(4), 355-373

Where does ensuring autonomous choice for individuals fit in as an appropriate goal for bioethics?

Autonomy is foundational to the field of bioethics, so one could reasonably hold that ensuring autonomous choice for individuals is an appropriate goal for bioethics as a field. As Ferguson et al. argue, "Agency, as a manifestation of autonomy, is foundational to human rights, and so to decent care because it establishes that 'quality' of human beings which demands they be acknowledged as individual persons and not merely as examples of a species."[28] The goal of ethical healthcare should be decent care which means that anything foundational to human rights and decent care would be foundational to the field of bioethics. I guess you can call it the transitive property of healthcare ethics.

Ferguson et al. carry their point about values, justice, and flourishing further by acknowledging that "the recognition of unique needs every individual has, and the *direct control and decision-making every individual* should be able to enact in the care she/he receives and how she/he receives it (emphasis added)."[29] This concept of control and decision-making is one of the basic principles of medical ethics and autonomy. Without paying attention to the individual needs of each patient and supporting the patient's control over decision-making we would be violating the basic tenets of bioethics.

The maintenance of autonomy also must be a focus of the entire bioethics field because if special attention is not paid to that aspect of care, then it would be even harder to account for variations in contexts. You can only have so many moving parts before the system begins to fail. In this case, by ensuring that patients are able to make autonomous choices,

---

28 Ferguson, J. T., Karpf, T., Weait, M., & Swift, R. Y. (2009). *Decent care: Living values, health justice and human flourishing*, p.11.

29 Ibid, p. 3.

we can build into that the need to account for the patient's particular life and situational contexts. Focus and attention always seem to bring about increased adherence.

One might very well wonder how healthcare workers should handle emergency situations where patients require the consent of community leaders to undergo lifesaving procedures. Context plays a significant role in answering that question. I say that because if the healthcare workers were active, vital members of the community and the community had specific cultural responsibilities, then those healthcare workers would assuredly have a familiarity of what to do in emergency situations. That familiarity might involve having a list of community leaders to contact or a standing order/local law that regulates healthcare work activities in those situations. This might particularly be true in Native American tribal locations where the tribe acts as an autonomous state and everyone would be like-minded about lifesaving procedures.

The situation would become more complicated if the patient was part of an unrecognized ethnic community that has no independent, autonomous government. In that case, the healthcare workers would most likely have no idea that the patient requires consent of community leaders prior to certain medical procedures or in certain lifesaving situations. This situation would be further complicated by the patient's mental status (conscious, unconscious, mentally incompetent) or ability to communicate desires/preferences. The bottom line decision of what action to take might fall to whatever best fits the fact that the patient presented to healthcare workers in an emergency situation with the implicit intent of being helped/healed to the greatest extent possible. In the absence of contextual clues or inputs, that choice should ethically meet the best intent of both the patient (to be healed) and the healthcare workers (to heal). What more can one expect in time-sensitive, emergency situations besides one's best, most sincere intent to help another human in need.

To circle back around for a second and clarify a point, I made some assumptions about the nature and definition of autonomy that other people might not similarly assume. I interpreted autonomy to be defined by the context of the people involved and not necessarily a set-in-stone absolute so that autonomy would have some built-in flexibility. If we default to a Western concept of autonomy with a focus on "self" to the exclusion of "non-self", then we will be in for some trouble. I think we do have the power to frame, or reframe as the case may be, the way we look at the question of autonomy to include the individual and the community and contextual variations or anomalies. That is one of the things about medical ethics that gives me a modicum of hope and encouragement…that we can debate, discuss, define and shape the philosophical basis for and practical application of ethics in not only the healthcare setting, but also the society as a whole.

Essay 1

Identity and Well-being

Introduction

A person's total well-being is an amalgamation of one's mental, physical, and emotional well-being and is intrinsically linked to one's identity and sense of self. The Mental Health Foundation considers emotional well-being essential to enabling a person "to function in society and meet the demands of everyday life" which when coupled with strong mental health allows a person to "have the ability to recover effectively from illness, change or misfortune."[30] The question arises as to which aspects of life have the greatest impact on one's identity and thereby have the greatest impact on well-being. One could correctly posit that one's identity is most strongly influenced by how one views oneself and is viewed by others within the context of one's ethnic community and how one adapts to changes to one's health and wellness.

Communal Context of Identity

As Blackhall et al. argue, one can be on a continuum of self-identity between being "autonomous agents whose dignity and worth come from the individual choices we make with our lives" and the result of "social web within which we exist."[31] Blackhall et al. further suggest that not only will different ethnic groups occupy different points on the continuum, but individuals within an ethnic group may also hold various points along the continuum based on the individual's experience and mores.[32] Communal context provides a foundation to establish one's identity. Whether one tends to one end of the continuum or the other end, one's identity is anchored by the communal context within which one lives which lends one strength and enhances one's well-being.

Adaptation to Impairment

Another factor that impacts one's identity is the way one handles and adapts to impairment and disease. Chronic illness and impairment can

---

30 BeLonG To. (2010). Retrieved from http://www.belongto.org/resource.aspx?contentid=4574

31 Blackhall, L. J., Frank, G., Murphy, S., & Michel, V. (2001). Bioethics in a different tongue: The case of truth-telling. *Journal of Urban Health, 78*(1), 59-71.

32 Ibid.

shift one's view of self and throw one's sense of identity into a state of chaos. As Charmaz posits, "chronic illness with impairment intrudes upon a person's daily life and undermines self and identity."[33] By undermining the sense of self and one's identity, impairment can have deleterious effects on one's well-being. Charmaz further suggests that "the body, identity, and self intersect in illness [and by adapting] to accommodate to physical losses and to reunify body and self ... in socially and personally acceptable ways."[34] Through the process of adapting to the changes the mind and body undergo during chronic illness, a person can gain strength of self and a renewed sense of identity. Anytime an individual is able to strengthen one's identity, she will gain well-being.

Conclusion

The two components of identity that have the greatest impact on well-being are the communal context within which one lives and the self-knowledge gained from adapting to illness and change. The communal context of one's life provides foundational identity that grounds and strengthens one. If an individual has a strong foundational identity, then one can more easily handle the traumatic changes caused by chronic illness and impairment. Then, by going through the process of adaptation, one gains even more strength of identity. In the end, one's well-being is enhanced and secured by the combination of the two components of identity.

---

33 Charmaz, K. (1995). The body, identity, and self: Adapting to impairment. *The Sociological Quarterly, 36*(4), 657-680.

34 Ibid, p. 658.

References

BeLonG To. (2010). Retrieved from http://www.belongto.org/resource.aspx?-contentid=4574

Blackhall, L. J., Frank, G., Murphy, S., & Michel, V. (2001). Bioethics in a differenttongue: The case of truth-telling. Journal of Urban Health, 78(1), 59-71.

Charmaz, K. (1995). The body, identity, and self: Adapting to impairment. The Sociological Quarterly, 36(4), 657-680.

Essay 2

HMONG AND RESPECT FOR AUTONOMY

Introduction

Anne Fadiman's book, *The Spirit Catches You and You Fall Down*, tells the tragic story of a young Hmong girl who was caught in the cultural chasm between Western medicine and Hmong philosophy of life. The young Hmong girl, Lia, suffered from epilepsy and septic shock which are both easily managed medical conditions. Unfortunately, Lia was a victim of the cultural disconnect between her caregiver Hmong parents and the Western physicians responsible for her treatment. Fadiman came to believe that Lia's "life was not ruined by septic shock or noncompliant

parents but by cross-cultural misunderstanding."[35] Fadiman drew a
clear portrait of a clash between the parents and the physicians based
on mutual misunderstanding due to language, cultural, and religious
differences. While the story centers on a specific situation, the lessons
learned can be a guide to understanding why one must consider cultural
context when evaluating the application of biomedical ethics. This paper
will address the idea that of the bioethics principles, respect for autonomy
as put forth by Beauchamp and Childress might have some valid meaning
to the Hmong given the lessons learned from Fadiman's story of Lia's
tragedy.

Respect for Autonomy

Beauchamp and Childress describe respect for autonomy as both a
negative and positive obligation. As a negative obligation, one must
ensure that an individual is not "subjected to controlling constraints by
others."[36] As a positive obligation, one must ensure "respectful treatment
in disclosing information and actions that foster autonomous decision-
making."[37] One important consideration in the Beauchamp and Childress
principle for respect for autonomy is the concept of self versus delegated
decision-making. In a UCLA study of 800 individuals of which two
hundred were Korean American, 200 Mexican American, 200 African
American, and 200 European American, Korean Americans and Mexican
Americans were more likely than African Americans and European
Americans to "believe that family should make the decision about the use

---

35 Charmaz, K. (1995). The body, identity, and self: Adapting to impairment. *The Sociological Quarterly, 36*(4), 657-680.

36 Beauchamp, Thomas L.; Childress, James F. (2013). Respect for Autonomy. *In Principles of Biomedical Ethics* (7th ed.). New York: Oxford University Press, p. 107.

37 Ibid.

of life support."[38] While the original investigators believed that the study showed an alternative to patient autonomy which the researchers termed a "family-centered model", Beauchamp and Childress believe that this is still an exhibition of individual autonomy.[39] As Beauchamp and Childress contend that, "even if the patient delegates that right to someone else, the choice to delegate can itself be autonomous."[40] The salient point coming out of this aspect of Beauchamp and Childress' principle is that an individual's autonomous decision can be derived from any source or multiple sources of information and advice. If a patient's culture requires the family to provide input and reach a consensus prior to making certain decisions, then the medical team should honor that process to maintain patient autonomy. The Western mind might perceive the family's input or involvement as coercive or divisive, but many cultures would view being forced to make a decision without that vital input as controlling and robbing them of their autonomy.

Beauchamp and Childress went on to discuss how the implications and impact that a conflict of culture can have on patient autonomy. Another study of how the Navajo values affect patient response to disclosure of risk and medical prognoses provided a powerful look into lessons healthcare providers can learn from the observation of others' cultural values and how providers can honor those values while maintaining patient autonomy. The Navajo cultural belief in the power of language "to shape reality and control events" gives healthcare providers invaluable insight into how they can take these lessons and build a richer, more inclusive concept of autonomy. The bottom line for Beauchamp and Childress is that healthcare providers have a professional obligation

---

38 Ibid, p. 109.

39 Ibid.

40 Ibid.

"to respect a person's autonomous choices, whatever they may be."[41] This obligation does not constrain a healthcare provider to the rigid, Western conception of patient autonomy, but rather includes the cultural variations and contexts that serve to make respect for autonomy a rich and dynamic bioethical principle.

Hmong Cultural Philosophy

Hmong culture is based on a patriarchal structure where "multiple extended families are organized into large closely knit communities known as clans" and the "well-being of the clan and the family take priority over the individual."[42] Furthermore, any medical decisions must be made by a clan elder of the male head of the household rather than solely by the individual.[43] Fadiman's story about Lia drew a clear picture of the conflicting cultural context between Western rationalism and Hmong animism contentiously crashing into each other to the detriment of a young girl, Lia, who was dependent upon the harmonious collaboration of these two realities for her wellbeing. Both realities failed to help her because of their mutual misunderstanding, suspicion, and prejudice of the other culture. Neither of the two sides of the situation realized that their "view of reality is just one view, not reality itself."[44] The doctors believed that the rationalistic Western medical view of the world was the only way to treat Lia. The doctors believed so strongly in their Western education and training

---

41 Beauchamp, Thomas L.; Childress, James F. (2013). Respect for Autonomy. *In Principles of Biomedical Ethics* (7th ed.). New York: Oxford University Press, p 110.

42 Thorburn, S., Kue, J., Levykeon, K., & Zukoski, A. (2013). "We don't talk about it" and other interpersonal influences on Hmong women's breast and cervical cancer screening decisions. *Health Education Research.* 28(5): 760–771. doi: 10.1093/her/cys115.

43 Ibid.

44 Fadiman, Anne. (1997) *The spirit catches you and you fall down: a Hmong child, her American doctors, and the collision of two cultures.* New York: Noonday Press, p. 276.

that they could not see the Lee's point of view. In typical Western medical fashion, the doctors also felt that paternalistic medicine would win the day and Lia's family would accept and appreciate the doctor's advice and help. The doctors had a hard time understanding the Hmong fear of common medical practices such as blood tests and surgery.[45]

The Lee's, on the other hand, could not imagine any other way of viewing the situation than through the lens of the traditional Hmong belief of animism. The Lee's looked at Lia's medical problem of epilepsy as soul loss rather than the Western diagnosis of epilepsy. Because each side saw a different cause for the malady, they each saw a different way of treating the problem. As Fadiman noted, the Lee's "version of reality fails to match that of their doctors pretty much across the board."[46] The Lees did not understand how or why to give Lia her medicine and the doctors did not know how to convince the Lees the medication was vital. The cultural conflict that contributed to Lia's condition could have been avoided if the medical doctors implemented Beauchamp and Childress' respect for autonomy.

Conclusion

Fadiman's book, The Spirit Catches You and You Fall Down, can be seen as a clarion call for greater implementation of cultural context in medical respect for autonomy. One would anticipate that as medical professionals implement respect for autonomy with the cultural context of the patient, then outcomes among minority and ethnic individuals might be increased. Beauchamp and Childress' respect for autonomy, due to its inclusive nature, would serve the Hmong people well when in healthcare situations.

---

45 Ibid.

46 Fadiman, Anne. (1998) *The spirit catches you and you fall down: a Hmong child, her American doctors, and the collision of two cultures*. New York: Noonday Press, p. 62.

References

Beauchamp, Thomas L.; Childress, James F. (2013). Respect for Autonomy. In Principles of Biomedical Ethics (7th ed.). New York: Oxford University Press

Charmaz, K. (1995). The body, identity, and self: Adapting to impairment. The Sociological Quarterly, 36(4), 657-680.

Fadiman, Anne. (1998) The spirit catches you and you fall down :a Hmong child, her American doctors, and the collision of two cultures New York : Noonday Press.

Thorburn, S., Kue, J., Levykeon, K., & Zukoski, A. (2013). "We don't talk about it" and other interpersonal influences on Hmong women's breast and cervical cancer screening decisions. Health Education Research. 28(5): 760–771. doi: 10.1093/her/cys115

Essay 3

ETHNOCENTRISM TO ETHNOPLURALISM: CHANGING PERSPECTIVES ON PATIENT AUTONOMY AND CULTURAL CONTEXT

Introduction

Bioethics is a field that has undergone tremendous growth and change over the last seventy years. Ever since the time of the Nuremberg Code in 1947 and the Belmont Report in 1978, bioethics has moved toward practices based on the principles of benevolence, non-maleficence, autonomy and justice. Of these four principles, the principle of autonomy can vary the most depending on the racial, cultural and enthographic gap between the patient and the medical providers. In order to bridge the gap, one must "appreciate the diverse value systems of ethnic minority groups, and understand how unexamined cultural assumptions by health professionals can underpin judgments of the quality and appropriateness of care."[47] Medicine and medical research in the US have been heavily influence by and predicated upon the mores and values of western society and culture. This Euro-centric focus has predominated the early practice of bioethics and the manner in which those principles are interpreted and applied to the practice of medicine. Ideally, the interpretation of autonomy within bioethics must take the racial, cultural and ethnographic context of the patient's situation into account so that medicine cannot only be practiced ethically, but also effectively. This paper will discuss how to redefine patient autonomy within an ethnographic context and why one can apply this globally to healthcare ethics.

Patient Autonomy

Autonomy in keeping with the general philosophy of bioethics has various theories about what the term actually means. Autonomy can be defined as "the capacity to act freely in making decisions in accordance with choices that have been determined by the individual, acting without interference from others."[48] The aforementioned definition can be refined by the addition of respect for an individual's autonomy as the

47 Sinclair, C., Smith, J., Toussaint, Y., & Auret, K. (2013). Discussing dying in the diaspora: Attitudes towards advance care planning among first generation Dutch and Italian migrants in rural Australia. *Social Science and Medicine, 101*, 92. doi: 10.1016/j.socscimed.2013.11.032

48 Ozolins, John; Grainger, Joanne. (2015). Foundations of Healthcare Ethics: Theory to Practice (p. 42). Cambridge University Press. Kindle Edition.

affirmation of an individual's "right to independently make choices" and perhaps more importantly, "[to] act according to their principles, values and beliefs, without coercion from others."[49][50] Beauchamp and Childress espouse a three-condition theory of intentionality, understanding and noncontrol that is focused on nonideal conditions instead of an ethereal ideal autonomy.[51] The malleability of Beauchamp and Childress' concept of autonomy is reliant upon including context so that the principles, values and beliefs of the individual can be taken into account. The patient's decision-making is dependent upon the patient's autonomy which is defined by the patient's ethnographic context.

Cultural Context—the Lottery

Cultural context should not be misunderstood as radical moral relativism or even radical cultural relativism as depicted in Shirley Jackson's "The Lottery." While Shirley Jackson intended "The Lottery" to be a commentary on American society's proclivity to blindly following traditions, one cannot help but see a similarity to the rituals practiced by the people of Pre-Colombian Mesoamerica and South America. The Maya, Inca, and Aztecs regularly sacrificed people, usually captured prisoners, but sometimes members of their own society (especially children), in order to control the weather and influence gods to favor them. The Lottery similarly sacrificed a member of their society in order to influence the harvest as Old Man Warner suggests when he says, "Lottery in June, corn

---

49 Beauchamp, T. L., Walters, L., Kahn, J. P. & Mastroianni, A. C. (2008). Contemporary issues in bioethics (7th ed.). Belmont, CA: Thomson Wadsworth.

50 Ozolins, John; Grainger, Joanne. (2015). Foundations of Healthcare Ethics: Theory to Practice (p. 40). Cambridge University Press. Kindle Edition.

51 Beauchamp, T. L. & Childress, J. F. (2013). Respect for Autonomy. In *Principles of Biomedical Ethics* (7th ed.). New York: Oxford University Press.

be heavy soon." I mention this to bring back the idea that the argument supporting The Lottery is cultural relativism which holds that all cultural beliefs are equally valid and that truth itself is relative, depending on the cultural environment. Therefore, the entire situation of the Lottery might be morally bereft in modern Western ideology, but for the people who live in the fictitious society of "The Lottery", all religious, ethical, aesthetic, and political beliefs are completely relative to the individual within that specific society. Again, this is not to say that radical cultural relativism should be employed in bioethics, but rather one should lean on constrained relativism.

This would serve to recognize and affirm the differences between cultures, but does not simply deem a practice or belief acceptable just because a group of people hold it to be so. As Arthur Kleinman argues, "one must compare alternative ethical formulations with the ethical standards he or she holds for the evaluation of a particular problem in a particular context."[52] The enthographic approach put forth by Kleinman requires medical providers to fully appreciate and engage with the "lived moral orientations" of their patients in order to minimize the influence of the Western ethical standards on situations where those standards are not valid.[53] This concept is especially important when considering medical care among patients of non-Western ethnicities because those cultures largely hold that the individual's autonomy is rooted in, and subservient to, social, familial, and communal obligations.[54] The medical provider must understand that the patient's autonomy must be viewed through the lens of the patient's ethnographic context.

---

52 Kleinman, A. (1995). Medicine, anthropology of. In W. T. Reich (Ed.), *Encyclopedia of bioethics* (3rd ed., pp. 1725-1730). London: MacMillan, p. 1729.

53 Ibid.

54 Ibid.

Cultural Context: Stranger in a Strange Land

The idea of ethnographic context is more like the Robert Heinlein novel *Stranger in a Strange Land* than Shirley Jackson's "The Lottery". Heinlein's protagonist, Valentine Michael Smith, is a human who was raised on Mars by Martians with no human contact for most of his life. Therefore, he was culturally and ideologically a Martian in thought, word and deed. Upon his return to the Earth, Smith was placed in Bethesda Hospital for observation and only attended by male staff because he had never seen a human female. One nurse, Gillian Boardman, was overcome with curiosity and, viewing her exclusion as a challenge, decided to sneak in to see Smith. During her visit with Smith, Nurse Boardman shared a glass of water with him. Nurse Boardman was unaware of Martian customs and by sharing the water unknowingly became a "water brother" which is considered a deep and profound relationship by the Martians. The situation in *Stranger in a Strange Land* is not dissimilar to the experience of a medical team when inadvertently stumbling through the cultural mores and belief system of a patient from an ethnic minority. Sometimes the best intentions might have serious, unintended implications that can have deleterious effects on patient care.

Cultural Context Applied to Patient Autonomy—Analysis

Context plays a critical role in the theory of autonomy as Beauchamp and Childress consider "the appropriate criteria for substantial autonomy are best addressed in a particular context."[55] Because Beauchamp

---

55 Beauchamp, T. L. & Childress, J. F. (2013). Respect for Autonomy. In *Principles of Biomedical Ethics* (7th ed.). New York: Oxford University Press, p. 105.

and Childress insist that context plays a role in determining autonomy, their theory of respect for autonomy can therefore be applied across a wide range of contexts. An example of this is the analysis Beauchamp and Childress present from the UCLA study of elderly subjects from different ethnic backgrounds (Korean American, Mexican American, African American, and European American) and the subjects' responses to questions about informed consent. In that study, Korean Americans and Mexican Americans were less likely than African Americans or European Americans to believe that a patient diagnosed with metastatic cancer should be informed of the diagnosis. This preference profile carries over to the preference for being informed of terminal prognoses and patient-centered decisions on life support decisions; the latter decision should be made by the family in the Korean American and Mexican American cultural contexts. The difference in application or interpretation of autonomy based on context does not invalidate the patient's autonomy in terms of understanding, intentionality, or non-control. By having autonomy based on the patient's individual context, the theory of respect for autonomy can be applied globally.

The main reason that Beauchamp and Childress's model can be applied across a multiplicity of contexts is because of their definition of the constituent parts of their model. Beauchamp and Childress's model for autonomy is a patient-sourced decision that not only includes intentionality, understanding, and noncontrol, but also includes the possibility that the patient's decision-making criteria are untethered from the standard Western ideas of autonomy as based in individualism, personal happiness, and self-actualization. Cultural differences need not hinder autonomy. Rather different cultural contexts, if understood and appreciated, serve to ensure patient autonomy and maintain the integrity of the informed consent process for clinical healthcare and biomedical research.

Cultural Context Applied to Patient Autonomy—the Art of Medicine

As Hippocrates has described medicine, "The art is long, life is short..." One can look at this as saying that learning the art or expertise of medical practice is not an easy journey. Recent advances in medicine have focused attention on an evidence-based medicine approach to healthcare that, while valuable, seems to undervalue ethnographic beliefs and traditional aspects of patient and family care. Surbone and Baider argue that "[t]he art, however, is subtle and ... is characterized, in part, by the ability to apply the science of medicine to the individual patient's unique illness, with particular attention to the nuances of social and familial circumstances and culture and of communication."[56] Medical providers must understand that individuals live in social situations and make choices based on context. Dependence on family or community may not diminish one's freedom of choice, but rather provide the confidence, support, and moral valuation that allows people to define and exercise autonomy. If medical providers consider how each person sees himself or herself in relation to others, then those same medical providers can view autonomy through a cross-cultural lens, rather than strictly through a scientific, clinical lens that strips away all cultural perspectives.

Conclusion

Bioethics and medical providers need to remain mindful that ethics and ethnographic competency must be taken and applied as an interwo-

---

56 Surbone, A. & Baider, L. (2013). Personal values and cultural diversity. *Journal of Medicine and the Person, 11*(1) 16. doi: 10.1007/s12682-013-0143-4

ven whole.[57] If a medical provider only views patient interactions and treatment plans through the lens of ethnographic and cultural sensitivity and fails to apply that within the framework of bioethics, then that medical provider is just as wrong as if she had ignored the patient's context. Both ethics and context must be considered equally so that medical providers can walk the fine line between honoring the patient's culture and the provider's ethical duties. One caveat to the application of ethnography to bioethics is, as Minkoff posits, "cultural sensitivity encompasses an understanding of and respect for the differing valuation that people give to various moral domains. However, physicians need not surrender either the right to offer direction and counsel when a patient's choices are perceived to conflict with her own best interests or the right to conscientious refusal when asked to be a party to potentially harmful acts merely because of the entreaties of those with conflicting cultural beliefs."[58] Nevertheless, one can quite ably globally apply cultural context to patient autonomy as defined by Beauchamp and Childress for the benefit of both the patient and bioethics. One area that warrants further investigation is how removal from the ethnographic context by time (second or third generation immigrant versus first generation immigrant) or distance (living outside the ethnic community with no family/community support) affects the patient's autonomy and decision-making.

---

57 Minkoff, H. (2014). Teaching ethics: When respect for autonomy and cultural sensitivity collide. *American Journal of Obstetrics and Gynecology, 210*(4) 298-301. doi: 10.1016/j.ajog.2013.10.876

58 Ibid, p. 300.

References

Beauchamp, T. L., Walters, L., Kahn, J. P. & Mastroianni, A. C. (2008). Contemporary issues in bioethics (7th ed.). Belmont, CA: Thomson Wadsworth.

Beauchamp, T. L. & Childress, J. F. (2013). Respect for Autonomy. In Principles of Biomedical Ethics (7th ed.). New York: Oxford University Press.

Heinlein, R. (1961). Stranger in a Strange Land. New York: G. P. Putnam's and Sons.

Jackson, S. (1948). The Lottery. The New Yorker. June 26, 1948.

Kleinman, A. (1995). Medicine, anthropology of. In W. T. Reich (Ed.), Encyclopedia of bioethics (3rd ed., pp. 1725-1730). London: MacMillan.

Minkoff, H. (2014). Teaching ethics: When respect for autonomy and cultural sensitivity collide. American Journal of Obstetrics and Gynecology, 210(4) 298—301. doi: 10.1016/j.ajog.2013.10.876

Ozolins, John; Grainger, Joanne. (2015). Foundations of Healthcare Ethics: Theory to Practice (p. 40). Cambridge University Press. Kindle Edition.

Sinclair, C., Smith, J., Toussaint, Y., & Auret, K. (2013). Discussing dying in the diaspora: Attitudes towards advance care planning among first generation Dutch and Italian migrants in rural Australia. Social Science and Medicine, 101, 86-93. doi: 10.1016/j.socscimed.2013.11.032

Surbone, A. & Baider, L. (2013). Personal values and cultural diversity. Journal of Medicine and the Person, 11(1) 11—18. doi: 10.1007/s12682-013-0143-4

Case Study

NT is an 8-year old, Vietnamese male who presents with flu-like symptoms. Upon physical review, the boy removes his shirt and you notice a pattern of very distinct bruises on the boy's torso. You ask

NT's mother about the source of the bruises, and she tells you that they are from a procedure she performed on him known as "cao gio." NT's mother explains that she performed cao gio to help NT recover from his illness and describes a process of lubricating NT's skin with massage oil and scraping along the skin with a coin in repeated, pressed strokes. NT's mother explains that cao gio is used to release unhealthy matter from the blood and improve circulation and healing. When you touch NT's back with your stethoscope, he winces in pain from the bruises.

Note: Cao gio originally came to Vietnam from China where it is known as Gua sha (刮 痧) and is widely practiced by people in Vietnam, Cambodia, Indonesia and other Southeast Asian countries and expatriate communities.

Ethical Questions to Ponder

(1) Should you contact Child Protective Services and report NT's mother? Why or why not?

(2) Does it matter that Olympic athletes voluntarily use similar practices like cupping to improve performance?

(3) What if NT's father was also there and he showed you that he had similar bruises because he had flu-like symptoms and the process healed him?

(4) When should a physician step in to stop a cultural practice?

(5) Would you think differently if you had a Vietnamese colleague who understood the practice of cao gio and characterized it as harmless?

Chapter 2

Justice and Justice for All...

One must distinguish between philosophical and legal approaches to justice when considering their application to healthcare ethics because the two areas are applied differently. Moreover, justice theory can be analyzed through the various paradigms of distributive justice, retributive justice, reparative justice, and structural justice. All of these factors affect justice and injustice in healthcare as pertains to healthcare resource allocation and practices.

What follows will be some discussion and argumentation focused on the foundational concepts underlying healthcare justice. Hopefully, the ground covered in this chapter will prompt some internal dialogue about how we as a society should view healthcare justice and how that justice could be implemented. You might even be encouraged to actively seek out avenues to positively impact the way healthcare justice is provided across your community.

Discussion Topics

What do we expect from the concept of justice when we apply it to healthcare?

When the discussion turns to expectations and theoretical speculation, I cannot help but wonder about the context and perspective of the person setting the expectations and speculating about various applications of those expectations. There can be a wide chasm between what "we" as healthcare providers expect justice in healthcare to entail versus what "we" as the American populace expect versus what "we" as the immensely diverse human species expect. While popular discussion covers some interesting aspects of justice in healthcare such as whether healthcare is special, or applying capability to distributive justice, or the wealth versus quality disparity, the aspect of the topic that intrigues me the most is the idea of context and the intersection of cultural competency in healthcare and social justice.[01 02 03 04]

The argument that the application of "critical consciousness [to healthcare]—which places medicine in a social, cultural, and historical context and which is coupled with an active recognition of societal problems and a search for appropriate solutions" will lead to social justice is compel-

01 Daniels, N. (2001). Justice, health, and healthcare. *American Journal of Bioethics 1*(2): 2-16, Spring 2001.

02 Emanuel, E.J. (2007). What cannot be said on television about health care. *Journal of the American Medical Association 297*(19), 2131-2133.

03 Kumagai, A. K. & Lypson, M. L. (2009). Beyond cultural competence: Critical consciousness, social justice, and multicultural education. *Academic Medicine 84*(6): 782-787.

04 Stone, J.R. & Rentmeester, C.A. (2015). Justice and the capability approach: Expanding distributive justice and connecting to structures.

ling.[05] The idea that there is a disconnect between multiculturalism and social justice that results in healthcare providers thinking that the pursuit of knowing the former will result in achieving the latter is startling and a call for introspection.[06] Often "we" as healthcare providers seem to approach social competencies like we approach biomedical competencies, we define cultural competency as acquiring "knowledge of characteristics, cultural beliefs, and practices of different nonmajority groups, and skills and attitudes of empathy and compassion in interviewing and communicating with nonmajority groups."[07] Critical consciousness and cultural competency are not simply gaining a finite level of knowing how particular groups act or think, or the skill to interact effectively with them, or even having a positive, receptive attitude when dealing with diverse groups. But rather, critical consciousness requires one to constantly undergo self-evaluation, education, and iteration to attain an awareness or consciousness of the interconnectedness of each of us and the world around us.

In order to treat each and every patient fairly, justly, and compassionately, we as healthcare providers must cultivate that cultural consciousness. Without that foundational quality, we might be hard pressed to treat patients, manage health systems, and develop public policy that provides social justice in healthcare.

I would have to say that we as healthcare practitioners need to become patient advocates in a different way than previous generations. First, on an individual patient basis we need to work in a collaborative way with social services workers and financial advocates and third party plan analysts to identify basic needs that the patient is lacking and the means to help

---

05 Ibid.

06 Kumagai, A. K. & Lypson, M. L. (2009). Beyond cultural competence: Critical consciousness, social justice, and multicultural education. *Academic Medicine 84*(6): 782-787.

07 Ibid, p. 783.

relieve those unmet needs. On the level of the health system or the society, we can help educate the policy makers about what areas need attention and how we, as a society, might be best able to remedy the ills of society that are causing the ills of its members.

Another area of concern is the potential impact of our environment and food choices (availability) on one's health status and the link to the social and economic status of the communities. An area that piques my interest is the limited healthy choices resulting from one's living conditions and location as referenced in the Unnatural Causes documentary. The amount of mental and physical stress on the body caused by living in a location that subjects one to air pollution, poor housing, lack of access to grocery stores, violence, and transportation that limits options even more is incalculable.

The access to grocery stores for people who live in large cities is of particular interest to me because during my internal medicine residency I lived in New York City and during my cardiology fellowship I lived in Philadelphia. Both of those cities are quite large and had an interesting grocery store dynamic. I did not get to see too much of the various boroughs in New York City because of the transportation and time constraints I had during my residency. I had to travel solely by public transportation and had very little free time, so I had to limit my shopping to locations close to work and home. Fortunately, I lived on the Upper East Side within walking distance from the hospital and had multiple grocery options because the area is very affluent, the residents demand fresh produce and other foods, and they are able to pay a premium that must be charged to offset the high real estate cost the business must pay. On the other end of the spectrum is North Philadelphia where I did my fellowship. The predominant demographic of that area is African-American and the area has extremely high rates of poverty, crime, drug use, and violence. Not surprisingly, there is also an extremely low number of grocery stores in the area. I was more fortunate than the people who lived in the community surrounding the hospital in North Philadelphia because I could afford to have a car and live in another section of Philadelphia that had more affluence, less crime, less drug use, and less violence. Not surprisingly, there were also more grocery stores in my neighborhood.

A final interesting note, I spent a lot of time in Philadelphia's Chinatown which is in the heart of the city about six or seven blocks from the Liberty Bell and Independence Hall. Chinatown was rife with crime and far from affluent, but there were at least seven grocery stores in a section that was four blocks by five blocks in size. It makes one wonder how we can change the social and living conditions in an area like North Philadelphia.

What are the uses and limitations of distributive justice theory and structural justice theory in thinking through problems of justice in healthcare?

For some, the discussion of the distributive model of justice begins by arguing that most views are too narrowly focused on distributive justice at the expense of other aspects of justice. American political theorist and feminist, Iris Young, notes a couple of problems with distributive justice. The first one is that the model would tend to limit the discussion of social justice to the allocation of material goods, such as things, resources, income, wealth, social position, and jobs.[08] According to Young, the preoccupation with material things would prevent us from considering the social structures and institutional contexts that cause the current pattern of distribution of such material goods. The second problem

---

08 Young, I. M. (2011). *Justice and the politics of difference*. Princeton, NJ: Princeton University Press. Displacing the Distributive Paradigm (pp. 15-38).

noted by Young is the tendency to stretch the discussion to include non-material goods and burdens, such as rights, power, opportunity, and self-respect.[09] Young argues that treating these non-material goods and burdens as something distributable, just like the material goods and burdens, would in the end distort their very nature. For example, once you look at power as something distributable, this would cause one to misunderstand that "power is a relation rather than a thing" and to miss the fact that power is "a structural phenomenon of domination."[10]

Young concludes by positing that whether social justice talks about material or non-material goods and burdens, the distributive model of justice is not sufficient to adequately handle all the various issues. This leads Young to proposing a structural justice model that works in coordination with distributive justice. Young feels that "a focus on the distribution of material goods and resources inappropriately restricts the scope of justice, because it fails to bring social structures and institutional contexts under evaluation.[11] The effects of structural injustice were shown by Levin and Schiller in their narratives about the CEO and the sharecropper. This highlights how the provision of justice can benefit from giving consideration to the social and class context of the individuals within the larger society. This contextual consideration fits nicely with Rechlin's discussion of solidarity with regard to social responsibility in healthcare. This can be thought of as "the disposition to take particular care of the needs and interests of the weaker members of the group."[12] One might see a striking similarity between that concept and Jesus' preaching good news to the poor (Luke 4:18), where He identifies Himself with the "least"

---

09 Ibid.

10 Ibid, p. 31.

11 Ibid, p. 20.

12 Reichlin, M. (2011). The role of solidarity in social responsibility for health. *Medicine Health Care and Philosophy, 14*, 365-370.

among men, and sets treatment of the poor as the criterion by which He will recognize His chosen ones (Matt. 25:31–46).[13] The structural and contextual existence of individuals and groups within society seems to be a crucial addition to the application of distributive justice to healthcare.

In which ways does a structural conception of justice (a la Young) challenge traditional liberal conceptions of autonomy?

In order to assess the ways in which a structural conception of justice challenges traditional liberal conceptions of autonomy, one can start with a foundational definition of liberal autonomy. Some ethicists posit that "[l]iberal conceptions of autonomy have always revealed an underlying general concept understood in terms of self-government, self-determination, or a kind of self-ownership of values, beliefs, desires, and choices."[14] Even though liberal autonomy can be thought of as atomistic and independent with the focus being the individual's perception of self, people are not necessarily able to dislocate themselves from the context of their lives. Young makes this point part of her discussion on the structural conception of justice when she argues that simply because we cannot separate ourselves from our history and affiliations we must look to structural justice as a way to evaluate an individual's pursuit of autonomy and real justice.

If society's members evaluate their autonomy within the context of their social and cultural histories and the manner in which that context has affected and shaped their development as people, then one will realize

---

13 Toth, W. J. (2007). Preferential option for the poor. In J. Varacalli, M. Coulter, & R. Myers (Eds.), *Encyclopedia of Catholic social thought, social science, and social policy: Vol. 2* (pp. 873-874). Lanham, MD: Scarecrow Press.

14 Ikonomidis, S. & Singer, P. A. (1999). 527 Autonomy, liberalism and advance care planning. *Journal of Medical Ethics 25*, (522) p. 522–527.

that one must think of oneself as part of ongoing communities, defined by reciprocal bonds of obligation, common traditions, and mores. This placement of the individual within the social context means that structure plays a critical role in justice that goes beyond what the traditional liberal conception of autonomy allows.

In light of considering structural justice as a revised view of autonomy, one must understand that this revised view does not obviate the issues raised by social structures and their incumbent injustices. Young lends the term "oppression" to the concept of structural injustices and clarifies "oppression" into the categories of exploitation, marginalization, powerlessness, cultural imperialism, and violence.[15] Oppression, as seen by Young, "is structural [and] its causes are embedded in unquestioned norms, habits, and symbols, in the assumptions underlying institutional rules and the collective consequences of following those rules."[16] We, as healthcare professionals, need to assess the existence of these norms, habits, and symbols that lead to oppression in our practice settings and our communities in order to make corrections in our practices to account for those factors. Cognizance is the first step to correcting an unhealthy environment and challenging the traditional concept of autonomy with a structural, contextual consideration of justice is a good way to start that process.

What are some of the ways in which healthcare workers can ensure justice for their patients?

The question as to how we as healthcare providers can ensure justice to our patients is the logical next step after determining the root cause of the injustice. For instance, if mental illness results in the loss of autonomy

---

15 Young, I. M. (1990). *Justice and the politics of difference*. Princeton, NJ: Princeton University Press. Five Faces of Oppression (pp. 39-65)

16 Ibid, p. 41.

secondary to lack of decision-making capability, then ensuring that the patient has a surrogate decision-maker in place who has the patient's best interest at heart would be paramount to ensuring justice for the patient. On the other hand, the driving force behind the injustice might be the lack of ability to adhere to a certain medication therapy because of their employment. Some regimens require the freedom to eat meals at certain times or use the restroom or the side effects impair functions directly related to the job. In those instances, we should make sure we understand the requirements of the regimen and ask probing questions so that we do not prescribe medication the patient cannot take. Ideally, we would be able to work with the patient to design medication therapies that fit their budget, their lifestyle constraints, and their healthcare needs. On a more global basis, we can discuss cases like that with our colleagues in order to raise awareness and share best practices for ensuring justice for our patients. As I noted previously, being aware of the issue and the injustices is essential because without that starting point we might not get to the second step of addressing the injustices.

When is representation a justice problem?

Bioethics places a great deal of emphasis on the four basic principles of beneficence, non-maleficence, autonomy, and justice. Part of the pursuit for patient autonomy and justice necessitates that the healthcare system acknowledges the cultural and ethnic requirements of patients and inculcate that information into the decision-making process. However, where does the onus for representation in healthcare lie? We can see how difficult dealing with exceptional patient situations can be through the lens of two case studies.

The first case we will consider is that of LJ, an elderly African American woman with a malignant melanoma on her foot, who refused medical treatment based on her faith. In this case, the hospital staff did not have experience dealing with such an extreme interpretation of Christian healing, so had difficulty understanding why the patient refused medical treatment that to an outward observer would seem quite logical.[17] This refusal was even more unexpected because LJ's belief system was not typical of a Pentecostal believer. The fact that LJ's children could not come to a unanimous agreement about how to support LJ made the situation that much more untenable for the hospital staff. Given that communication with the patient was breaking down rapidly and the patient's family had better insight into the patient's belief system than anyone else, one would logically determine that the hospital staff should have asked the family for guidance about how best to interact with the patient. Also, the patient's family should have seen that their mother was shutting down and stepped in to help defuse the situation before it escalated out of control. Should we have expected the patient to be self-aware and request a member of her church's clergy act as a mediator or even a teacher about the patient's beliefs for the medical team?

The second case we will consider, about a young Sudanese woman with HIV, was complicated because there are not many Sudanese immigrants in the United States. Therefore, experience dealing with that culture in America is not as pervasive as experience with other cultures. Also, the young woman was unwilling to have "interpreters into the room because she does not trust them to keep her HIV status confidential."[18] As the Sudanese woman was withdrawing from care, should the medical team have been able to acknowledge their lack of knowledge about the woman's belief systems and cultural mores and seek out someone who could

---

17 Powell, T. (1995). Religion, race, and reason: The case of LJ. *Journal of Clinical Ethics,* 6(1), 73-7.

18 Rentmeester, C.A. and DeLancey, D.B. (2008). Trust, translation, and HAART. *Hastings Center Report, 38*(6), 13

explain the woman's decision-making process and ways to improve communication? One has to wonder how much responsibility lies with the patient and how much lies with the medical providers to bridge a communication or understanding gap. Men often joke that women expect them to be mind-readers. In order to avoid needing to read our patient's minds, we need to implement systemic structures that identify situations in which patients' needs are not being fully represented and implement steps to remedy the situation.

The task of explaining LJ's belief system to the ethics committee should reside with the medical team because at the end of the day the medical team is responsible for not only identifying any barriers to diagnosis and treatment, but also finding ways to overcome those barriers. Now, this is not to say that the patient has no responsibility in this situation. I believe that if a patient wants to have autonomy, then she needs to take ownership of her care and articulate when she is not being heard. Unfortunately, patients may not be able to identify the communication barrier and bridge the gap. For that reason, I suggest that the healthcare system treat a patient's religious and cultural belief systems the same way we treat a foreign language. Ideally, the ethics committee should have people who have an intimate understanding of various religious and cultural beliefs and can act as an "interpreter" for the patient. We as healthcare providers have no qualms about asking for a medical consult from another physician when the patient's disease state is outside the range and scope of our practice. We should feel equally comfortable saying, "I need help understanding what this patient is telling me because I do not understand the context of their life. Please help me understand so I can help this person."

The real work needs to be done by rolling up our sleeves and taking concrete action. Part of that action is to push back against intolerance when you see it, invest time and money in hearing marginalized voices and perspectives, and work to be inclusive in your own life. We can lead by example. All it takes is the strength of will and character to see it through to the end.

Also, while I agree with Young's contention "that equality as the participation and inclusion of all groups sometimes requires *different* treatment for oppressed or disadvantaged groups" (*emphasis added*),[19] *different* does not mean blanket favoritism. I would personally feel like less of a person if I received a benefit I did not earn because of my race or gender. To borrow a bit of proverbial wisdom, "Give a man a fish, and you feed him for a day. Teach a man to fish, and you feed him for a lifetime." We need to support the growth and development of the disenfranchised and not give them handouts and treat them as children who cannot fend for themselves.

How do cultural imperialism and violence express as justice problems in healthcare?

Maybe my view of this is oversimplified, but cultural imperialism and violence seem to fall under the category of structural justice versus structural violence. The idea of imposing one set of cultural beliefs and standards on an entire society with complete disregard for the different cultural beliefs of individual groups or members within the society should be considered unjust.

Structural cultural imperialism leads to many of the societal woes as discussed in the Unnatural Causes video entitled "Bad Sugar" when investigating the plight of the Native American tribes. The cultural diet and manner of living life was stripped away and replaced with a governmentally-supplied diet. The Native American population took the various

---

19 Young, I. M. (2011). *Justice and the politics of difference*. Princeton, NJ: Princeton University Press.

ingredients and tried to do the best they could to make the food work in their culture. One example is the use of flour, lard, and oil to make and fry some pastry-like dietary staple. Unfortunately, the nutritional profile of the diet combined with the other cultural changes to the Native American lifestyle created the perfect storm for diabetes to run rampant through the community.

The Native population has no way to combat many of the cultural changes that destroyed their diet and their lifestyle. As S. Leonard Syme pointed out in the "Bad Sugar" video, those ethnic populations that have been dispossessed of their lands and their history have no way of reclaiming them. He goes on to postulate that those populations that are "ripped from their roots" have a higher incidence of disease because of the cultural imperialism that they experience.

One of the results of the subjugation of the Native American population has been economic and educational barriers that further exacerbate the healthcare issues. The educational opportunities and consequently the financial future of the population is almost non-existent. Economics has been shown time and again to play a significant role in the structural and distributive justice of health across a society. By ignoring the Native American culture and imposing another culture on the Native American population, the society as a whole has displayed cultural imperialism and violence that results in unjust distribution of healthcare across the population.

One might be tempted to over compensate for the cultural imperialism and suggest that the Native American population should return to their cultural roots in order to improve their diet. This premise would be supported by research that points to "specific loci in the DNA of some Native Americans that affect their insulin sensitivity." However, I believe that the cause of the dietary and health fiasco among the Native American population is not so much because they deviated from their tradition diet, but more so because the replacement welfare food welfare they receive is "in the form of packaged and processed starches, seed oils, and low fat animal sources—foods that have potentially contributed to increasing metabolic syndrome in the US population more generally." Originally, Native Americans were not solely hunter-gatherers, but rather relied on a combination of hunting-gathering and cultivation of crops. Their lifestyle was also much more active and allowed them to burn through the carbohydrates more easily than their current sedentary lifestyle. That food sourcing and lifestyle was destroyed by the appropriation of their lands and the forced welfare system imposed by the federal government.

Ideally, the Native American population would be given the financial, educational, technical support, and encouragement to completely reinvent their way of life. One of the key transitional factors would be helping them understand the correlation between their cultural heritage and their health. By showing the nutritional components of their historical, cultural diet and offering ways to reobtain that diet, the Native American population might be stirred to throw off the yoke of their poor federally provided welfare diet in favor of more traditional foods or nutritionally equivalent alternatives. After that, they should be provided with the financial means and knowledge to grow their own crops that meet that new dietary requirement. Also, the federal government should increase the financial support to the tribes so that they can obtain locally and regionally sourced nutritious food around the reservation that they cannot grow or supply themselves. Lastly, the tribes should be given support and guidance to develop better educational systems and economically viable industries so that they have a path to future growth and self-sufficiency. Give a man a fish and he eats for a day, teach a man to fish and he eats for a lifetime. It is time to remind the tribes they knew how to fish and help them do it again.

How ought the interests of marginalized populations and minoritarian perspectives be represented to promote justice in healthcare?

The idea of how one ought to do something regarding others always makes me think of the Golden Rule, "do unto others as you would have them do unto you." Unfortunately, that adage might not allow enough flexibility to accommodate the wants and needs of different people with different preferences. When considering how one ought to treat marginalized and minority populations in an attempt to promote healthcare justice, one would need to identify which differences of situation are morally relevant. Ideally, one would hope that healthcare providers would ignore any internal prejudice against a patient's race, ethnicity, or medical conditions when deciding how to act towards that person. Also, one would hope that those same healthcare providers would consider how the patient's situation might lead to that patient receiving less healthcare equity or justice than other patients might receive.

In the documentary, *Out of the Shadow*, the struggles Millie encountered when trying to obtain effective treatment for her schizophrenia within the healthcare system exemplified how healthcare justice can be elusive even when the patient and the patient's family are actively trying to find some.[20] The psychological trauma that the younger daughter suffered because of Millie's undiagnosed and, later, poorly treated illness was evident throughout the documentary. The daughter called her mother by her given name of Millie or Mildred and never called her "Mom" or even the less familiar form of "Mother". The trauma may have also lead to the decision to lie to Millie in order to obtain consent for medical treatment. What was Millie's daughter's motivation? If we question the decisions

---

20 Smiley, S. (2004). Out of the shadow. Vine Street Pictures.

made by a family appointed guardian of a person with a mental disorder, can we trust anyone to act purely in pursuit of healthcare justice for someone who might be at risk for unjust treatment?

Furthermore, is the healthcare system set up to adequately treat those with mental disorders? Millie was in and out of institutions for the majority of her adult life with little success and no long-term solutions until Millie was entered into a non-traditional treatment program. Oliver Sacks referenced the residential communities that sprang from the "asylums and therapeutic farm communities of the nineteenth century" that foster "community, companionship, opportunity for work and creativity, and respect for the individuality of everyone there... coupled with the best of psychotherapy and whatever medication is needed." Unfortunately, even though those institutions have positive outcomes, there are only enough to accommodate a few hundred patients and cost more than $100,000 per patient per year.[21] How does this serve justice when the best therapeutic option is only available to less than 1% of the patient population? Sometimes a more expensive therapeutic intervention actually saves money in the long run. Maybe using therapeutic communities for those with mental disorders is one of those situations where we are better off spending more money upfront for better outcomes and potentially decreased expense in the future.

The implementation of residential therapeutic communities would potentially decrease the homeless population by upwards of 20 to 25%, if the National Coalition for the Homeless' estimate of the number of homeless with some form of severe mental illness is correct.[22] In 2006, a National Mental Health Association study showed that supported hous-

---

21 Sacks, O. (2009). (2009). The lost virtues of the asylum. *The New York Review of Books, LVI*(14), 50-52.

22 Ibid.

ing that includes "mental health treatment, physical health care, education and employment opportunities, peer support, and daily living and money management skills training" is effective for treating the mentally ill. Supported housing programs or residential therapeutic communities are more likely to help homeless people with mental illnesses to recover and achieve residential stability than psychotherapy and medicine without community engagement.

The easiest way to reintroduce and implement this type of program would be in a government funded, longitudinal, randomized, controlled study that compares the residential therapeutic community to mental health treatment alone with no other support and to mental health treatment with housing but without any other community support features. The government would need to be the main funder of this study because the greatest benefit would be a societal benefit of fewer homeless who are economically more productive. Secondarily, pharmaceutical manufacturers might be interested if the study would show increased compliance to medication therapy which would increase manufacturer profits.

The ethics of undocumented immigrants and healthcare

As a nation, we Americans seem to be caught in a never-ending debate about immigration—particularly undocumented or illegal immigrants. The rigorous debate about immigration in general only becomes more intense when the discussion turns to the impact on social programs such as education and healthcare. In 2006, the Department of Homeland Security estimated that there were 11.6 million undocumented immigrants in the U.S. The obstacles to medical care experienced by undocumented immigrants are both structural, a reflection of their disadvantaged position in the labor market, and political, the result of public policies to reduce costs and to mitigate the potential of social services to attract more migrants.

When one adds end of life care to the immigration-healthcare distribution debate, the ethical picture becomes incredibly complicated and
contentious. Across the board, end of life care accounts for a disproportionate amount of total healthcare expenditure. On average, we spend
more money on the last decade of life than we spend during our lives
from birth to that point. Undocumented immigrants are more likely than
U.S. citizens and documented immigrants to be uninsured and therefore
healthcare costs will be borne by U.S. citizens and the healthcare systems.
One of the major questions that needs to be addressed is, how do we
ethically distribute limited healthcare resources and obtain healthcare
justice for undocumented immigrants facing end of life care? There is a
great deal of rancor about immigration in general, so resolving how to
get Americans to pay for expensive end of life care for people who many
believe should not even be here will be an ethical and political minefield.

How do theories of justice motivate responses to injustices in healthcare?

Injustices in healthcare, as Dr. Martin Luther King, Jr. stated in a
speech on human rights in 1966, is "the most shocking and inhumane...
of all forms of inequality." The responses to disparities and injustices in
healthcare operate through many levels of influence including the patient,
provider, organization, community, and government policy. By working with those actors and within those structures, one can start to affect
change that addresses those injustices.

In order to evaluate those injustices, one needs to employ "a moral
lens—that can better discern the value-laden questions" that arise in the

field of bioethics.[23] That moral lens is the coordination of the various theories of justice that create a mental and philosophical mindset to evaluate situations in one's environment. Whether the theory one employs is Rawlsian ethics or Kantian ethics, distributive justice or structural justice, cultural competence or cultural consciousness, etc., the simple act of considering the theories of justice causes one to try to apply those theories in both real and imagined situations. Once the process of evaluating ethical situations begins, one will be inclined to continue to consider various theories of justice when confronted with injustices in healthcare. Therefore, theories of justice motivate responses to injustices in healthcare by creating a questioning, inquisitive mental state and the framework within which one can evaluate the injustice.

References

Daniels, N. (2001). Justice, health, and healthcare. American Journal of Bioethics 1(2): 2-16, Spring 2001.

Emanuel, E.J. (2007). What cannot be said on television about health care. Journal of the American Medical Association 297(19), 2131-2133.

Kumagai, A. K. & Lypson, M. L. (2009). Beyond cultural competence: Critical consciousness, social justice, and multicultural education. Academic Medicine 84(6): 782-787.

Stone, J.R. & Rentmeester, C.A. (2015). Justice and the capability approach: Expanding distributive justice and connecting to structures.

Levin, B. W., & Schiller, N. G. (1998). Social class and medical decisionmaking: A

---

23 Rubin, D. (2010). A Role for Moral Vision in Public Health. *Hastings Center Report*, *40*(6):20-22.

neglected topic in bioethics. Cambridge Quarterly of Healthcare Ethics, 7, 41-56.

Reichlin, M. (2011). The role of solidarity in social responsibility for health. Medicine Health Care and Philosophy, 14, 365-370.

Toth, W. J. (2007). Preferential option for the poor. In J. Varacalli, M. Coulter, & R. Myers (Eds.), Encyclopedia of Catholic social thought, social science, and social policy: Vol. 2 (pp. 873-874). Lanham, MD: Scarecrow Press.

Young, I. M. (2011). Justice and the politics of difference. Princeton, NJ: Princeton University Press. Displacing the Distributive Paradigm (pp. 15-38).

Ikonomidis, S. & Singer, P. A. (1999). 527 Autonomy, liberalism and advance care planning. Journal of Medical Ethics 25, (522) p. 522—527.

Young, I. M. (1990). Justice and the politics of difference. Princeton, NJ: Princeton University Press. Five Faces of Oppression (pp. 39-65)

Keelty, C. (2016, November 12). Dear White people, your safety pins areembarrassing. Huffington Post. Retrieved from http://www.huffingtonpost.com/entry/dear-white-people-your-safety-pins-are-embarassing_us_58278b9de4b02b1f5257a36a

Powell, T. (1995). Religion, race, and reason: The case of LJ. Journal of Clinical Ethics, 6(1), 73-7.

Rentmeester, C.A. and DeLancey, D.B. (2008). Trust, translation, and HAART. Hastings Center Report, 38(6), 13-14.

Young, I. M. (2011). Justice and the politics of difference. Princeton, NJ: Princeton University Press.

Unnatural Causes, California Newsreel, 2008. Episode 4 "Bad Sugar"

National Coalition for the Homeless. (2009). Mental illness and homelessness. http://www.nationalhomeless.org/factsheets/Mental_Illness.pdf

National Mental Health Association. (2006). Ending homelessness for people with mental illnesses and co-occurring disorders. Retrieved from http://www.nmha.org.

Sacks, O. (2009). (2009). The lost virtues of the asylum. The New York Review of Books, LVI(14), 50-52.

Smiley, S. (2004). Out of the shadow. Vine Street Pictures.

Mendola, A. (2014). Undocumented and at the end of life. Narrative Inquiry in Bioethics, 4(2), 179-184.

Rubin, D. (2010). A Role for Moral Vision in Public Health. Hastings Center Report, 40(6):20-22.

Essay 4

ECONOMIC INEQUALITIES AND SOCIAL INJUSTICE VIEWED WITHIN THE RUBRIC OF STRUCTURAL AND DISTRIBUTIVE JUSTICE

Introduction

Richard Wilkinson offers compelling and thought-provoking insight in his TED Talk about how economic inequalities harm societies. Wilkinson's talk examines the comparative effect of income disparity within a society across democratic market-driven nations as opposed to the standard consideration of the impact of Gross Domestic Product (GDP) or Gross National Product (GNP) to compare one society to another. However, Wilkinson's talk also does not specifically consider the effect of economic inequalities on access to healthcare or health status inequalities. Nevertheless, Wilkinson's discussion of mental illness, violence, and social mobility allows one to gain insight into understanding the relationship between justice and healthcare. This paper will consider those three discussion points in the context of understanding the relationship between justice and healthcare and present three other concepts that would help augment

Wilkinson's discussion in terms of racial and ethnic inequalities in access to healthcare and health status inequalities suffered by those with mental illnesses.

Mental Illness

Wilkinson not only compared data among various developed nations across the globe, but he also compared data across the fifty United States. Within that analysis, Wilkinson first considered WHO data that used "the same diagnostic interviews on random samples of the population to allow us to compare rates of mental illness in each society."[24] The data showed that among developed nations there was a three-fold difference in the number of individuals with mental illness within each population with a corresponding linear relationship to economic inequality.[25] While the data are correlational and not causational, there is still a strong indication that where one finds great economic disparities, one is certain to find mental illness disparities. Those people with mental illness are subjected to further inequities in healthcare status and provision.

When one considers the history of mental illness in America, it is important to note that many mentally ill were pushed out onto the streets after many state-run mental hospitals were closed which led to a homeless population of mentally ill who are "a non-autonomous population granted full responsibility for their lives: responsibility without autonomy."[26] Advocates for the mentally ill often thought that psychiatric facilities

24 Wilkinson, R. (2011, July). *Richard Wilkinson: How economic inequality harms societies*. Retrieved from http://www.ted.com/talks/richard_wilkinson

25 Ibid.

26 Gaylin, W., & Jennings, B. (2003). Autonomy gone bonkers: The mentally impaired. In *The perversion of autonomy: coercion and constraints in a liberal society* (pp. 189-212). Washington, DC: Georgetown University Press.

were inhumane and coercive which obviates the basic tenet of auton-omy.[27] However, because the homeless mentally ill have no medical or ancillary psychiatric treatment, they are actually subjected to a decreased health status, both overall and compared to the rest of society, than they experienced when in the facility. This can be viewed as structural injustice for the mentally ill that results from the way that society views, values, and treats the mentally ill. Therefore, the economic inequality across society is correlated to increased mental illness which in turn contributes to unequal health status as a result of structural injustices. The injustice suffered by the mentally ill can be remedied in part by "recognizing [that the needs of the mentally ill] do not deny them respect as person; on the contrary, it is society's failure to recognize their special needs and vulner-abilities that is dehumanizing to the mentally impaired."[28] Once society recognizes and addresses those special needs by changing societal struc-ture, the mentally ill will have a better chance of obtaining the necessary health status required for improved healthcare outcomes.

Violence

A second area that Wilkinson addresses in his talk that can be applied to the relationship between justice and healthcare is violence. Wilkinson compares the level of violence in the American states with the Canadi-an provinces. Wilkinson's data analysis shows that a strong correlation exists between economic inequalities and the number of homicides in a society and the number of people incarcerated in a society. In fact, the difference is ten-fold between the poor and the wealthy for both per cap-

---

27 Gaylin, W., & Jennings, B. (2003). Autonomy gone bonkers: The mentally impaired. In *The perversion of autonomy: coercion and constraints in a liberal society* (pp. 189-212). Washington, DC: Georgetown University Press.

28 Ibid, p. 191.

ita homicides and incarcerations.[29] Wilkinson attributes the disparity not only to crime rates, but mainly to "more punitive sentencing, harsher sentencing. And the more unequal societies are more likely also to retain the death penalty."[30] The systemic violence is not limited to crime and punishment. The rate at which children drop out of high school is also directly related to the economic disparity within the society. One can infer from the data analysis presented by Wilkinson that economic inequality can produce social injustice and transitively, thereby cause healthcare inequalities.

The effect is more dramatic for the minority populations across America because those individuals are the most likely to be victims of homicide, commit homicide or violent crimes and be incarcerated in American prisons.[31] Violence is "a phenomenon of social injustice, and not merely an individual moral wrong, [because of] its systemic character, its existence as a social practice."[32] Wilkinson adds to this understanding of the impact on health by positing that "psychosocial effects of inequality" are caused by "threats to self-esteem or social status in which others can negatively judge your performance."[33] Iris Young adds another layer of granularity with her argument that "the oppression of violence consists not only in direct victimization, but in the daily knowledge shared by all members of oppressed groups that they are liable to violation, solely on account

---

29 Wilkinson, R. (2011, July). *Richard Wilkinson: How economic inequality harms societies*. Retrieved from http://www.ted.com/talks/richard_wilkinson

30 Ibid.

31 Lowery, W. (2016 July 11). Aren't more white people than black people killed by police? Yes, but no. Washington Post. Retrieved from https://www.washingtonpost.com/news/post-nation/wp/2016/07/11/arent-more-white-people-than-black-people-killed-by-police-yes-but-no/

32 Young, I. M. (2011). *Justice and the politics of difference*. Princeton, NJ: Princeton University Press.

33 Wilkinson, R. (2011, July). *Richard Wilkinson: How economic inequality harms societies*. Retrieved from http://www.ted.com/talks/richard_wilkinson

of their group identity."[34] An understanding of the impact of economic inequalities on systemic violence targeted at specific racial groups helps to elucidate the consequent deleterious impact on healthcare inequalities.

Social Mobility

The third aspect of Wilkinson's talk that draws a correlation between economic inequality and social injustice is social mobility. Wilkinson's analysis of income data between generations showed that there is "actually a measure of mobility based on income. And at the more unequal end, fathers' income is much more important — in the U.K., U.S.A., and in Scandinavian countries, fathers' income is much less important. There's more social mobility."[35] This concept has dramatic implications for those in America at the lower end of the socio-economic scale because people born to parents in the lower bracket are more likely to remain in the lower bracket and have sustained, "inherited" economic inequality and the incumbent social injustice. One can readily see how economic and social injustice derived from social immobility can carry over to healthcare injustice and inequalities due to both the lifestyle attached to the social status and society's perception of the individual.

In an attempt at humor, Wilkinson quips that "if Americans want to live the American dream, they should go to Denmark."[36] Over the last century, that statement has become increasingly true for the vast majority of America. In her discussion of oppression and social division of labor, Young notes "that in the nineteenth century the doctrine of equal

---

34 Young, I. M. (2011). *Justice and the politics of difference.* Princeton, NJ: Princeton University Press.

35 Wilkinson, R. (2011, July). *Richard Wilkinson: How economic inequality harms societies.* Retrieved from http://www.ted.com/talks/richard_wilkinson

36 Ibid.

opportunity had a more radical and democratic meaning than it does now. Then it meant that there were no barriers to material and social improvement to those who would work hard and develop their skills. Equal opportunity meant everybody who worked hard could be somebody".[37] The opportunities across the American business landscape have dwindled in the last century which has resulted in less social mobility and more social injustice. Young goes on to argue that "the propertied basis of [professional] positions remains a crucial determinant of class division and class struggle in our society; social conflict to a large degree concerns access to the exclusive professional positions that carry entitlements to goods and social power."[38] One of the contributing factors that plays a role in this social dynamic is the fact that "job structure in the United States is divided between prestige positions for which certification is difficult and costly to acquire, and a vast array of low-skill, low-wage, low-mobility positions that carry little autonomy and creativity."[39] The lack of autonomy is an element of structural injustice that leads to oppression. Young considers the targeting of menial labor to minorities "as a form of racially specific exploitation" which she places within the context of a distributive model of justice.[40] The distributive model of justice can help to solve many ills of social injustices, but the simple redistribution of wealth or goods cannot reverse all of the injustices of exploitation as long as "institutionalized practices and structural relations remain unaltered."[41] One of the key mechanisms to establishing justice in the face of exploitation is to implement "reorganization of institutions and practices of decision making,

---

37 Young, I. M. (2011). *Justice and the politics of difference*. Princeton, NJ: Princeton University Press, p. 214.

38 Ibid.

39 Ibid, p. 215.

40 Ibid, p. 51.

41 Ibid, p. 53.

alteration of the division of labor, and similar measures of institutional, structural, and cultural change."[42]

What about Cultural Influences?

Wilkinson's presentation could have been enhanced by addressing the cultural and racial differences among the various countries that may contribute to the way differences in economics impact societies. For instance, how does an individualistic society differ from a collectivist society? Individualistic cultures, such as the United States, place a great deal of emphasis on personal identity and self-determination. On the other hand, collectivistic cultures, such as African, Asian and Middle Eastern societies, emphasize the value of belonging, and as a result, majority influence happens to be greater.[43] How would that factor impact Wilkinson's analysis of the data? Wilkinson mentions that Japan and Sweden have similar per capita net income, but arrived at that point through different means. Japan has more equal wages and equal taxes across society, whereas Sweden has highly differentiated wages and an extremely progressive tax rate so that each group has a similar net income and standard deviation of net income across their societies.

Conclusion

Wilkinson's TED Talk about social ills stemming from economic inequalities is a starting point to consider the impact of social injustice on racial and ethnic healthcare inequalities and health status inequalities in the mentally ill. That discussion can be augmented by intertwining those

---

42 Ibid.

43 Sadat, H. (2011). Social psychology: A glimpse of social conformity through the ages. *In Motion*. Retrieved from http://www.inmotionmagazine.com/hrcr11/hsadat2.html

ideas with the concepts presented by Iris Young's discussion of structural injustices, oppression, and systemic exploitation. Mental illness, violence, and social mobility can be placed within the rubric of structural and distributive justice to arrive at a clear understanding of the factors that influence healthcare injustice and to elucidate methods to address those injustices.

References

Gaylin, W., & Jennings, B. (2003). Autonomy gone bonkers: The mentally impaired. In The perversion of autonomy: coercion and constraints in a liberal society (pp. 189-212). Washington, DC: Georgetown University Press.

Lowery, W. (2016 July 11). Aren't more white people than black people killed by police? Yes, but no. Washington Post. Retrieved from https://www.washingtonpost.com/news/post-nation/wp/2016/07/11/arent-more-white-people-than-black-people-killed-by-police-yes-but-no/

Sadat, H. (2011). Social psychology: A glimpse of social conformity through the ages. In Motion. Retrieved from http://www.inmotionmagazine.com/hrcr11/hsadat2.html

Wilkinson, R. (2011, July). Richard Wilkinson: How economic inequality harms societies [Video file]. Retrieved from http://www.ted.com/talks/richard_wilkinson

Young, I. M. (2011). Justice and the politics of difference. Princeton, NJ: Princeton University Press.

Essay 5

Undocumented Immigrants and End-of-life Care: the Search for Healthcare Justice

Introduction

People have been moving from one country to another throughout history in search of a better life, more opportunity, or a more promising future. A person who enters a different country for the express purpose of establishing permanent residence is an immigrant. Immigrants can be divided into three general categories based on the method of immigration: legal immigrants who are sponsored by family or employers, refugee or asylum-seeking immigrants who are avoiding persecution, and undocumented immigrants who are in the country illegally. An undocumented immigrant can be one who has illegally entered the country or one who legally entered the country, but had a status change such as visa expiration, asylum denial, or fraudulent citizenship application. The response of nations to these immigrants can have dramatic impact on the lives of the immigrants and the social structure of the nation receiving them. When Africans entered the North African Spanish-held autonomous cities of Ceuta and Melilla in the 1990s in an attempt to immigrate to the European Union and escape political turmoil and economic strife in their homelands, the asylum-seeking immigrants were denied and became undocumented immigrants who struggled economically and with healthcare.[44] On the other hand, over 100,000 Cuban refugees were expelled from Cuba in the 1980s during the Mariel boatlift and in the 1990s during the rafter crisis and granted refugee status in the US which allowed them greater access to healthcare than received by the undocumented African immigrants received in the European Union.[45] Healthcare access and resultant health status of undocumented immigrants is compromised because they are less likely to have healthcare insurance and are not eligible for coverage under the Affordable Care Act (ACA). Diminished access results in less preventive care and often delays in seeking care when needed which leads to worse morbidity and mortality rates for chronic diseases than the national average. The impact is even greater when the disease state requires end-of-life care and allocation of limited healthcare resources. Combining all three factors (undocumented immigrants, end-of-life care, and allocation of limited healthcare resources) leads to an immense crisis of medical and social ethics. This paper will discuss the healthcare crisis faced by undocumented immigrants facing end-of-life care and ways to ethically distribute limited healthcare resources and obtain healthcare justice for undocumented immigrants facing end-of-life care.

Undocumented Immigrants—by the Numbers

According to statistics from the Department of Homeland Security, as of 2008, there were an estimated 11.6 million undocumented immigrants

---

44 Martinez, O., Wu, E., Sandfort, T. et al. (2015). Evaluating the impact of immigration policies on health status among undocumented immigrants: A systematic review. *Journal of Immigrant and Minority Health, 17*(3), 947-970. doi:10.1007/s10903-013-9968-4

45 Ibid.

in the US of which 81% were from Latin America.[46] [47] The states of California, Texas, Florida, New York, New Jersey and Illinois account for over 60% of unauthorized immigrants which can place a heavy burden on the healthcare infrastructure of those states.[48] Undocumented immigrants comprise just over 5% of the American workforce and annually add about $12 billion in taxes.[49] Even with their contribution to the tax rolls, undocumented immigrants do not qualify for the ACA and most have no healthcare insurance and must pay for care out of pocket. Most primary healthcare is provided to them through community clinics and hospital emergency departments. Ironically, oftentimes those facilities lack adequate staffing and equipment in general because they are usually poorly funded and serve a large patient population. Moreover, those facilities often have a lack of culturally and linguistically trained staff to handle the variety of undocumented immigrants. Because the undocumented immigrants are less likely to receive preventive care, they are "more likely to delay seeking necessary care, and have worse chronic disease morbidity and mortality as a result."[50] The higher rate of chronic disease morbidity and mortality results in a greater number of undocumented immigrants facing end-of-life care with poor access to healthcare services.

---

46 Ortega, A. (2015). When politics trumps health: Undocumented Latino immigrants and US health care. *Medical Education Cooperation with Cuba, 17*(4), 1. Retrieved from http://www.scielosp.org/pdf/medicc/v17n4/1555-7960-medicc-17-04-0059.pdf

47 Sanchez, G. R. & Sanchez-Youngman, S. (2013). The politics of the healthcare reform debate: Public support of including undocumented immigrants and their children in reform efforts in the U.S. *International Migration Review, 47.* p. 442 - 473. doi:10.1111/imre.12027

48 Ortega, A. (2015). When politics trumps health: Undocumented Latino immigrants and US health care. *Medical Education Cooperation with Cuba, 17*(4), 1. Retrieved from http://www.scielosp.org/pdf/medicc/v17n4/1555-7960-medicc-17-04-0059.pdf

49 Ibid.

50 Ibid, p. 1.

End-of-life Care

End-of-life care can cover a vast array of disease states and patient populations. Some patients might have disease states such as cancer that might be end-of-life care, but through treatment the patient is cancer-free and the treatment, while expensive, is not truly end-of-life care. For this paper, end-of-life care will be considered a chronic disease state, such as End Stage Renal Disease (ESRD) that requires ongoing or intensive treatment to prolong life or increase the patient's quality of life. A thorough understanding of the needs of the undocumented immigrant population with ESRD requires being able to estimate the number of undocumented immigrants with ESRD and the cost of their medical care as well as the factors that impact their care. These data are difficult to uncover simply because of the nature of that population being undocumented immigrants. Much of the analysis relies on using theoretical data extrapolated from anecdotal case studies such as Annette Mendola's case study of Henri, an undocumented Haitian immigrant with ESRD. Using Henri's case as the basis for analysis, one can develop an appreciation for the decisions that healthcare providers and society must face when developing ethical ways to distribute just healthcare to that patient population.

ESRD—Treatment Modalities, Cost, and Consequences

The primary treatment for patients with ESRD is hemodialysis which comes with an annual price tag of approximately $72,000 per patient.[51] This cost is largely covered for all US citizens who qualify for

51 Raghavan, R. & Nuila, R. (2011). Survivors -- dialysis, immigration, and U.S. law. *The New England Journal of Medicine, 364*(23), 2183-5.

Medicare or Medicaid with ESRD through the End Stage Renal Disease program passed by Congress in 1973. Unfortunately for undocumented immigrants, the US passed the Consolidated Omnibus Budget Reconciliation Act (COBRA) in 1986 which "explicitly prohibits the use of federal funds for covering undocumented residents for nonemergency services such as dialysis."[52] This means that in most US states the burden of paying for long-term dialysis therapy for undocumented immigrants with ESRD who cannot afford to pay for their own care falls on the shoulders of tax payers.

Unfortunately, the lack of a structured, comprehensive dialysis program for undocumented immigrants coupled with the lack of opportunity for locating viable donors, results in ESRD patients resorting to getting their care in emergency departments. Additionally, those patients must also wait for ESRD complications to arise in order for their condition to be considered emergent and thereby qualifying for care in the emergency department.[53] In a small study done at Elmhurst Hospital Center in Queens, New York, Linden et al. found that 9% of undocumented immigrants with ESRD in their study had come to the US with a prior diagnosis of kidney disease expressly because they needed dialysis.[54] In the same study, 89% of patients would remain in the US if nothing changed in their health status or treatment plan in order to continue receiving kidney disease treatment. This means that those patients would continue to receive barely enough care to keep them alive, but at an inflated price and with poorer outcomes compared to other treatment options such as transplant.

---

52 Ibid, p. 2184.

53 Linden, E., Cano, J., & Coritsidis, G. (2012). Kidney transplantation in undocumented immigrants with ESRD: A policy whose time has come? *American Journal of Kidney Diseases, 60*(3), 354-359.

54 Ibid.

Research has shown that kidney transplant is superior to dialysis in terms of cost and outcomes including morbidity, mortality, and quality of life. Considering that a patient who receives "an organ from a living donor results in significantly greater transplant and patient survival at all stages of follow-up, the younger age of undocumented immigrants and their fewer comorbid conditions would make them ideal patients for successful transplant."[55] While the Organ Procurement and Transplantation Network of the US Department of Health and Human Services has specific policies in place for foreign nationals to enter the US temporarily for organ transplant surgery, there is no written policy covering undocumented immigrants. Generally, the lack of medical insurance covering transplant costs presents an insurmountable barrier excluding undocumented immigrants from transplant.

The vast majority of patients (96%) in the Elmhurst study indicated they would like to get a kidney transplant, but could only contribute $18,775 to the procedure.[56] With an average cost of $262,900 per kidney transplant billed by transplant centers in the United States in 2011, the balance of the cost would need to be absorbed by governmental entities or social programs. Ironically, even though the initial cost of the transplant and the post-operative care exceeds the yearly cost of dialysis, transplantation actually saves money over time. With estimates of an annual expense of more than $77,000 per patient for transplant versus $27,000 per year per patient for post-transplant maintenance therapy, transplantation would start to show cost-savings within two to four years.[57]

---

55 Ibid, p. 358.

56 Ibid.

57 Ibid.

Medical Ethics Considerations

The discussion of cost-savings connotes that the obligation or duty to provide care is a given in the equation even though the patient is an undocumented immigrant. On one hand, taking a broad view on the issue, one that ensures everyone receives the healthcare they need, regardless of their immigration status, would be a significant way to start instilling justice into the healthcare equation. As McCormick points out, employing a feminist theory of bioethics and justice would serve society well because "feminists call for a fuller grasp of the relational, social and interdependent character of persons, and for a recognition of the wider obligations of care and compassion for those in need."[58] A feminist ethic does not concern itself with whether a person is a citizen, immigrant, or undocumented immigrant, but rather that we are all humans, we all become sick, and we all need healthcare at some point in our lives.

The duty to provide care rests with the individual healthcare provider who is actively treating the patient. Because healthcare providers do not set policy or write laws, they must take smaller measures to ensure healthcare justice for undocumented immigrants. If one strips away the labels and looks solely at the patient, then one can readily see that undocumented immigrants are not so different from US citizens who are homeless or unemployed or lack medical insurance. Ideally, healthcare providers should welcome patients of all ethnicities and immigration statuses by encouraging cultural competency training that promotes human solidarity. By advocating for the underserved, disenfranchised patient populations, healthcare providers will be able to make strides toward increasing healthcare justice and equity received by those groups.

---

58 McCormick, P.T. (2003). Whose justice? An examination of nine models of justice. *Journal of Religion & Spirituality in Social Work: Social Thought* 22(2), 7-25.

On the national level, immigration politics in the US has become a point of contention across the entire society. In fact, immigration reform was one of the major issues debated in the 2016 Presidential election, just as the impact of immigration was debated during the 2009 federal healthcare reform.[59] The contention of opponents of healthcare reform was that undocumented immigrants would increase the cost of health care. Healthcare providers, politicians, health system policy makers, and others should work together with the goal of developing policy solutions based on healthcare justice, equity, and human solidarity.

Conclusion

The care received by undocumented immigrants with ESRD in the US has been less than effective and less than just. Injustices in healthcare, as Dr. Martin Luther King, Jr. stated in a speech on human rights in 1966, is "the most shocking and inhumane... of all forms of inequality". The responses to disparities and injustices in healthcare operate through many levels of influence including the patient, provider, organization, community, and government policy. By working with those actors and within those structures, one can start to affect change that addresses those injustices. In order to evaluate those injustices, one needs to employ "a moral lens - that can better discern the value-laden questions" that arise in the field of bioethics.[60] That moral lens is the coordination of the various theories of justice that create a mental and philosophical mindset to evaluate situations in one's environment. The simple act of considering

---

59 Sanchez, G. R. & Sanchez-Youngman, S. (2013). The politics of the healthcare reform debate: Public support of including undocumented immigrants and their children in reform efforts in the U.S. *International Migration Review, 47*. p. 442 - 473. doi:10.1111/imre.12027

60 Rubin, D. (2010). A Role for Moral Vision in Public Health. *Hastings Center Report, 40*(6), 20-22.

the theories of justice causes one to try to apply those theories in both real and imagined situations. Once the process of evaluating ethical situations begins, one will be inclined to continue to consider various theories of justice when confronted with injustices in healthcare. Therefore, theories of justice motivate responses to injustices in healthcare by creating a questioning, inquisitive mental state and the framework within which one can evaluate injustice. The healthcare community needs to apply this process to the provision of medical care for undocumented immigrants and maybe one day we will employ a broader-view approach to the problem and develop more just policy.

References

Aldridge, M. D. & Kelley, A. S. (2015). The myth regarding the high cost of end-of-life care. American Journal of Public Health, 105(12), 2411-2415. doi: 10.2105/AJPH.2015.302889

Campbell, G., Sanoff, S. & Rosner, M. (2010). Care of the undocumented immigrant in the United States with ESRD. American Journal of Kidney Diseases, 55(1), 181-191.

Chavez, L. (2012). Undocumented immigrants and their use of medical services in Orange County, California. Social Science & Medicine, 74(6), 887-893. doi: 10.1016/j.socscimed.2011.05.023

Garrido, M. M., Balboni, T. A., Maciejewski, P. K., Bao, Y., & Prigerson, H. G. (2015). Quality of life and cost of care at the end-of-life: The role of advance directives. Journal of Pain and Symptom Management, 49(5), 828-835. doi: 10.1016/j.jpainsymman.2014.09.015

Linden, E., Cano, J., & Coritsidis, G. (2012). Kidney transplantation in undocumented immigrants with ESRD: A policy whose time has come? American Journal of Kidney Diseases, 60(3), 354-359.

Martinez, O., Wu, E., Sandfort, T. et al. (2015). Evaluating the impact of immigration policies on health status among undocumented immigrants: A systematic review. Journal of Immigrant and Minority Health, 17(3), 947-970. doi:10.1007/s10903-013-9968-4

McCormick, P.T. (2003). Whose justice? An examination of nine models of justice. Journal of Religion & Spirituality in Social Work: Social Thought 22(2), 7-25.

Mendola, A. (2014). Undocumented and at the end-of-life. Narrative Inquiry in Bioethics, 4(2), 179-184.

Ortega, A. (2015). When politics trumps health: Undocumented Latino immigrants and US health care.

Medical Education Cooperation with Cuba, 17(4), 1. Retrieved from http://www.scielosp.org/pdf/medicc/v17n4/1555-7960-medicc-17-04-0059.pdf

Raghavan, R. & Nuila, R. (2011). Survivors -- dialysis, immigration, and U.S. law. The New England Journal of Medicine, 364(23), 2183-5.

Rubin, D. (2010). A Role for Moral Vision in Public Health. Hastings Center Report, 40(6), 20-22.

Sanchez, G. R. & Sanchez-Youngman, S. (2013). The politics of the healthcare reform debate: Public support of including undocumented immigrants and their children in reform efforts in the U.S. International Migration Review, 47. p. 442 - 473. doi:10.1111/imre.12027

Case Study

Isabel is a 16-year-old undocumented immigrant who has been followed at a regional pediatric heart center since age five for single-ventricle Fontan physiology. She lives with her parents and three siblings in a rural community, where her parents work as agricultural laborers. Isabel and two of her siblings immigrated to the Unites States as children and are, therefore, eligible for the Deferred Action for Childhood Arrivals

(DACA) program. Isabel's youngest sibling was born in the United States and is an American citizen.

Isabel's heart condition is now complicated by protein-losing enteropathy, tricuspid regurgitation, and decreased cardiac function. Her cardiologists have diagnosed her with end-stage heart disease and believe she will require a cardiac transplant to survive to adulthood. Due to her anatomy, Isabel is at a higher risk of a poor outcome if transplantation is pursued, and this risk will increase as her condition worsens. She is not a candidate for a ventricular assist device. After a discussion of the risks and benefits of a transplant, Isabel and her parents have indicated that they would like to pursue heart transplantation.

The cardiac transplantation team considers Isabel an acceptable candidate for transplantation despite her increased risk. However, the team has raised concerns about whether Isabel's status as an undocumented immigrant will adversely affect her ability to obtain the health care and medications required to maintain her long-term health following the transplant. Her first surgery was performed in Mexico, but subsequent surgeries have been performed at the regional pediatric institution. The regional children's hospital has committed to providing care and medications until Isabel reaches age 21, but the team has expressed concern about whether she would be able to afford the necessary care and medications after that point.

Ethical Questions to Ponder

(1) What roles should justice and fairness play and what roles do they play in the distribution of medical resources?

(2) How is that dynamic altered by the fact that organs are a scarce,

limited, national resource, donated by the population, that by law do not have a monetary value?

(3) What are the implications of excluding patients based on ability to pay?

(4) Does Isabel's potential inability to afford medical care past the age of 21 (which makes her more likely than the average transplant recipient to lose the graft) change the way the scarce organ should be allocated? Why?

(5) In what ways is assessing a patient's future (insurance, compliance, behaviors) a slippery slope for determining and addressing a current medical need?

Chapter 3

Research—Lessons from Tuskegee

Research ethics are the principles that govern the standards of conduct for medical researchers. Anyone involved in medical research must adhere to ethical principles in order to protect the dignity, rights and welfare of research participants.

To this end, all research involving human beings should be reviewed by an ethics committee to ensure that the appropriate ethical standards are being upheld. Ideally, the ethical principles of beneficence, nonmaleficence, justice and autonomy should be central to ethics committee discussions during ethical review.

Additionally, an examination of the core ethical issues in biomedical research involving human participants, especially vulnerable populations and communities, must consider a review of ethical, policy, and programmatic responses. One must also examine community-based research, informed consent, multinational research, genomics, and neuroscience in order to appreciate the breadth of the issue.

Discussion Topics

Ethics and the USPHS Syphilis Study at Tuskegee

The Tuskegee Syphilis Study was fraught with ethical issues, some of which had dire consequences for the relationship between the medical profession and the African-American community. The study seriously eroded the trust of the African American community towards the medical establishment. The damage done by the study was particularly damaging because it began during the economic wasteland of the Depression, which had left the blacks in the South especially destitute, and continued through the Civil Rights movement when blacks were fighting for equality. Those struggles made the African American community particularly distrustful of the federal government. Some commentators believe that there is evidence that African Americans did not seek treatment for AIDS in the early 1980s because of distrust of health care providers.

Aside from the obvious ethical issue of failure to gain informed consent from the study subjects, one of the worst examples of ethical malfeasance is the withholding of treatment for research purposes. Patient welfare was consistently sacrificed for the prospect of greater, more robust study data. Even though there was the federal mandate of the Henderson Act in 1943 for the reporting and treatment of venereal diseases, the PHS managed to find a way to avoid treating the study participants. The PHS went so far as to withhold penicillin treatment after the drug came to the forefront of treatment during WWII under the reasoning that no data were available proving the efficiency of penicillin treatment in late syphilis. The PHS researchers unilaterally determined that the benefits of non-treatment outweighed the benefits of treatment.

By withholding treatment from the known diseased patients, the study researchers acted with complete disregard for any basic ethical or moral propriety. While the impact to the study subjects and their families is quite obvious, the impact on the psyche of the African American community has been pervasive and long lasting. In some ways, the African American community has remained hesitant to seek medical attention and often doubts the validity of diagnosis and treatment to this day.

Paternalism, Federal Research Regulations, and the Belmont Report

Alan Wertheimer in his book, *Rethinking the Ethics of Clinical Research*, addresses some fundamental questions surrounding the field of medical research ethics, where the regulatory arena and a history of scandals like Nuremburg and Tuskegee combine to frame a great deal of debate and conjecture. The question of paternalism is one of those areas of debate that arises in Wertheimer's book.

Among many topics, Wertheimer specifically covers paternalism from multiple vantage points. Wertheimer first discusses the difference between the application of paternalism to clinical medicine and the application of paternalism to clinical research. Wertheimer considers clinical medicine to be anti-paternalistic because of the general consensus that a competent adult patient has the autonomy to reject treatment even if the physician thinks the patient is mistaken.[01] He breaks the analysis of paternalism down into points of comparison such as: indirect vs. direct, soft vs. hard, and individual vs. group.

Wertheimer then puts forth "a four-fold thesis."[02] The four parts of the thesis are "(1)the regulatory system for human research is paternalistic at

---

01 Wertheimer, A. (2011) *Rethinking the ethics of clinical research*. New York, NY: Oxford University Press.

02 Ibid, p. 20.

its core and (2)is a form of group soft-paternalism, [that] (3)may be perfectly justifiable, and (4)is compatible with the values that the principle
of informed consent is designed to serve even though research regulation
does not rely exclusively on the mechanism of informed consent."[03]

Wertheimer goes on to state that the Institutional Review Boards that
pre-determine whether a study is even permissible in the first place does
that through group soft paternalism. He believes "that the structure of
the system and many of the criteria that IRBs are asked to apply are best
justified by group soft paternalism."[04] That belief is highly consistent
with the Belmont Study published by the United States Department of
Health and Human Services in 1979. The Belmont Study considered
the ethical treatment of human study subjects in research. The Belmont
Study looked at the ethical principles of respect for persons, beneficence,
and justice and their subsequent practical application in research studies.

Both Wertheimer and the Belmont Study contend that the human
subject of the study should have informed consent, be given complete
information that can be comprehended, and should be participating
voluntarily. Moreover, they are in concurrence that the study subject and
society should have a net benefit from participation in the research study
with the majority of the benefit going to the study participant. Finally,
selection of the study participants for risky research should not be targeted from socially or individually disadvantaged groups (such as incarcerated, mentally infirm, poor, children, etc.).[05] If the research is beneficial
and not risky, then the study should be offered to all and not only those
favored by the researchers.

In essence, Wertheimer gave more depth to the discussion of ethics on

03 Ibid.

04 Ibid, p. 30.

05 *The Belmont Report*. Retrieved from http://www.hhs.gov/ohrp/humansubjects/guidance/
belmont.html

research studies presented in The Belmont Study. He gave a thorough and thoughtful analysis of the concept of paternalism from various perspectives that further elucidated the points laid out in the HHS report.

Ethics and Community-based Research, Equipoise and Research

Ernest Wallwork, in his article "Ethical Analysis of Research Partnerships with Communities," attempts to "identify the main ways of thinking ethically about the obligations of investigators and the roles and rights of communities in scientific research" through a review of the ever-growing literature on the subject.[06] In the analysis, Wallwork purports that the "advocates of community-partnership research implicitly adopt one of three models or paradigms for thinking ethically: application and specification; extension; and postmodern."[07] Within each of these three models, Wallwork highlights the key discussion points, pros and cons, and principles for applying the model to research. Quite often, this analysis requires a comparison of research ethics when applied to research among individuals with the standard usually being The Belmont Report and the Common Rule. As Wallwork's article is fairly comprehensive and wide-ranging, I will focus on the principle of social justice as it applies to community-based research and how it compares to the treatment of justice in The Belmont Report.

Wallwork notes that The Belmont Report mandates the protection of "vulnerable populations from exploitation and other forms of injustice" which is often copied by researchers and applied to community-based research.[08] However, while The Belmont Report's concept of justice fo-

---

06 Wallwork, E. (2008). Ethical analysis of research partnerships with communities. Kennedy Institute of Ethics Journal, 18(1), 57-85.

07 Ibid, p. 62.

08 Ibid, p. 71.

cuses on protecting individual subjects (children, prisoners, or indigent) from exploitation, the report considers the community population of these individuals as just that, an aggregation of individuals and not a collective entity. Wallwork uses the example that when The Belmont Report considers vulnerable populations such as welfare workers and prisoners, there is no thought of communities such as the Navajo having distinctive ethnic features and histories which may subject the community to receiving unfair treatment as a group.

The concept of distributive injustice carries over nicely from The Belmont Report's characterization of an individual subject to the application on a group or community level. Wallwork uses the example from a National Bioethics Advisory Commission report of clinical trials for treatment of malaria among the Malawi population. After the study showed that melfoquine is a superior drug for treatment, the Malawi people, as much as twenty years later, still failed to have the drug made available to them.[09] A strict interpretation of the Belmont Report might determine that there was only distributive injustice for the research subjects who had been part of the study, who received a less effective drug that did not cure the disease completely and left some organisms hiding in the liver; those subjects did not later receive the melfoquine.

There is a definite similarity in the treatment of social justice between that described by Wallwork with regard to community-based research and described by The Belmont Report with regard to individual research subjects. The similarity ends as The Belmont Report fails to consider the possibility that an historical group or community might have distinctive symbols, rituals, narratives, values, and institutions that bind them to-

---

09 NBAC. National Bioethics Advisory Commission. 2001. Ethical Policy Issues in International Research: Clinical Trials in Developing Countries. Volume 1: Report and Recommendations of the National Bioethics Advisory Commission. Bethesda, MD: NBAC. Available at http://bioethics.georgetown.edu/nbac/pubs.html

gether and might make them vulnerable to exploitation, whether intentional or not.

Randomized clinical trials (RCT) present an interesting collection of ethical dilemmas for the physician researcher. The primary ethical problem stems from one of the points that supposedly makes the study valuable—the randomized assignment of study participants to a particular arm of the trial. Most clinicians look to randomized, placebo-controlled, double-blind studies as the gold standard for clinically relevant information. However, since physicians are expected to give their patients the best available therapy, there becomes a conflict when their patient is involved in a research trial. One must wonder if the patient is still a patient or a research subject or some awkward combination of patient/subject. Enter the idea of equipoise, which is an attempt to find some ethical balance between the roles of physician and researcher. Unfortunately, there is little concurrence of opinion about the use and value of equipoise as applied to clinical research. Four types or theories equipoise have been suggested: individual equipoise (IE), clinical equipoise (CE), patient equipoise, and community equipoise. Charles Fried developed and has been the primary advocate for individual equipoise which stipulates that a physician may offer trial enrollment to her patient only when the physician is genuinely uncertain as to the preferred treatment. On the other hand, clinical equipoise, which was originated by Benjamin Freedman, requires that there exists a state of honest, professional disagreement in the community of expert practitioners as to what is the preferred treatment.

These two concepts seem to be the primary competing concepts regarding ethics of clinical trial participation. One might argue that individual and clinical equipoise offer separable and, by themselves, incomplete support for conducting clinical trials. IE focuses on the fiduciary responsibilities of the physician to patient in research trials. CE pushes for social approval of research by institutional review boards. In this sense IE and

CE are not necessarily competing concepts, but rather are complementary in nature.

Having said that, IE is the form of equipoise that should guide clinical research instead of CE guiding the research. One reason is the flaws that riddle the CE concept, such as the fact that CE confuses the ethics of clinical research with the ethics of medical care. Since RCT are not a form of therapy, but are first and foremost research study, there are no longer physician-patient relationships to maintain. Therefore, trying to apply the ethics of what a physician would do in clinical practice should have no bearing on what should be done in a research trial. The focus should be on how to ethically randomize or assign patients to one arm or another of a research trial.

Children and Non-beneficial Research

Society has a responsibility to provide protection for vulnerable populations involved in research studies. Vulnerability for an individual can be due to conditions that cause a person to have diminished capacity to make fully informed decisions for him or herself. Also, a population as a whole may be deemed vulnerable due to circumstances that leave the population susceptible to coercion or undue influence to participate in research projects. Children would be vulnerable due to their lack of ability to make decisions. The ethics of children participating in clinical research becomes more debatable when the research offers the children involved no clinical benefit. As a mother and physician, I guess I have divided loyalties about this topic, but I believe that the greater good warrants the inclusion of children in research even if there is no direct clinical benefit to the child.

The federal government has promulgated regulations in 45 CFR 46 that afford some protection for those groups, including Subpart D: Additional Safeguards for Children in Clinical Trials.[10][11] The federal regulations are further subdivided into four categories of permissible research involving children. Of the four categories, two categories address the more controversial areas of research with greater than minimal risk and no direct benefit to the child.

The regulations permit research if "the research presents experiences to subjects that are reasonably commensurate with those inherent in their actual or expected medical, dental, psychological, social, or educational situations" and if "the research is likely to yield generalizable knowledge about the subjects' disorder or condition which is of vital importance for the understanding or amelioration of the subjects' disorder or condition."[12][13] Both of these categories of research require consent of both parents or legal guardians "unless one parent is deceased, unknown, incompetent, not reasonably available, or does not have legal responsibility for the custody of the minor."[14] This requirement is stricter than the one parent requirement for research involving minimal risk or with direct benefit to the child. Also, the requirement for review by "the Secretary of the U. S. Department of Health and Human Services, after consultation with a panel of experts and following an opportunity for public review and comment" would highlight the enhanced concern for the safety and

---

10 Human Subjects Research. Code of Federal Regulations. (21 C.F.R. 53-4). (2009). Retrieved from http://www.hhs.gov/ohrp/humansubjects/guidance/21cfr53.html

11 Human Subjects Research. Code of Federal Regulations. (45 C.F.R. 46-7). (2009). Retrieved from http://www.hhs.gov/ohrp/humansubjects/guidance/45cfr46.html

12 Human Subjects Research. Code of Federal Regulations. (21 C.F.R. 53-4). (2009). Retrieved from http://www.hhs.gov/ohrp/humansubjects/guidance/21cfr53.html

13 Human Subjects Research. Code of Federal Regulations. (45 C.F.R. 46-7). (2009). Retrieved from http://www.hhs.gov/ohrp/humansubjects/guidance/45cfr46.html

14 Ibid.

welfare of children as research subjects.[15] [16]

Some might argue that the parents might fall into a vulnerable category and therefore might be unduly coerced into involving their child in research that less vulnerable parents might not permit. Theoretically, the involvement of an IRB and the DHHS would obviate the potential for that occurring. For a child to be inappropriately involved in a research study, multiple actors who are completely disparate from one another would need to simultaneously forsake their fiduciary obligations. The chance of that happening is so remote that one would necessarily conclude the protections to the child and the benefit to society are sufficient to support the participation of children in research even if the child received no direct benefit.

Institutional Review Boards

An Institutional Review Board (IRB) is a committee established to review and approve research involving human subjects and to ensure that the research be conducted in accordance with all federal, institutional, and ethical guidelines. The Food and Drug Administration (FDA) and the Department of Health and Human Services (DHHS) both stipulate that an IRB is an "appropriately constituted group that has been formally designated to review and monitor biomedical research involving human subjects...and protects the rights and welfare of those human research subjects."[17] The DHHS, however, barely touches on the concept of the independence of the IRB in their Institutional Review Board Guidelines.

----

15 Human Subjects Research. Code of Federal Regulations. (21 C.F.R. 53-4). (2009). Retrieved from http://www.hhs.gov/ohrp/humansubjects/guidance/21cfr53.html

16 Human Subjects Research. Code of Federal Regulations. (45 C.F.R. 46-7). (2009). Retrieved from http://www.hhs.gov/ohrp/humansubjects/guidance/45cfr46.html

17 http://www.fda.gov/RegulatoryInformation/Guidances/ucm126420.htm

The Guidelines indicate that the "IRB also functions independently of but in coordination with other committees. The IRB, however, makes its independent determination whether to approve or disapprove the protocol based upon whether or not human subjects are adequately protected."[18]

In its 2001 report on research involving human participants, the National Bioethics Advisory Commission (NBAC) uses the term "independent" in its recommendation 2.1: "The federal oversight system should protect the rights and welfare of human research participants by requiring ... independent review of risks and potential benefits."[19] Interestingly, none of the guidelines require the committee that reviews ethical aspects of research to be independent of the institutions where the research is carried out. Instead, they mainly address the independence of IRB members from the investigators or research project under review.

One might say that an intra-institutional review is independent if the IRB members are not principal investigators or collaborators of the research under review. In a stricter definition, IRB members must not be in the same academic or clinical department as the researchers. And in the strictest sense, the IRB members should not be part of the same institution, research center, or even university as the researchers conducting the research. Potential bias can exist when colleagues are reviewing each other's research proposals, but each individual IRB member has to decide on her own if she is free from bias, and decide how to address the bias if there is any.

An alternative is to use a commercial or non-institutional review board. While this would obviate possible collegial or institutional bias, this

18 http://www.hhs.gov/ohrp/archive/irb/irb_chapter1.htm

19 National Bioethics Advisory Commission. (2001). Ethical and Policy Issues in Research Involving Human Participants. Bethesda, Md.: National Bioethics Advisory Commission. Bethesda, MD: NBAC. http://bioethics.georgetown.edu/nbac/pubs.html

opens the process to undue influence from the drug manufacturer who would be the source of payment for the IRB. The IRB may be susceptible to a conflict of interest because they have a financial interest in keeping the drug company happy. This conflict of interest is the type of information that must be disclosed by anyone involved in the research process or involved in presenting or advocating for a particular therapy or treatment. There is no clear cut path to realizing an absolutely independent IRB, but the current process has been successful so far and should remain so as long as there is transparency in the process and due diligence when considering the value of a study.

A disconnect exists between protection of the individual versus protection of the community. Protection of the individual from a physical standpoint is much easier to determine than protection of the culture and values of the community as a whole. Not that protection of the community is unimportant, but rather there are significant barriers to effectively executing a postmodern paradigm in practice.

I have read some opinions about current research that does not adequately represent the community and I am not sure if people feel that the inadequate protection of the community is a lack of knowledge or an overt attempt to take advantage of a vulnerable community. I personally believe that the vast majority of researchers and IRB members operate in good faith effort to protect research participants and to be respectful to the community at large.

I think at the end of the day, one needs to acknowledge that the process of conducting community-based research can never reach a point of absolute theoretical perfection. Rather, I think one must consider each community-based study as an opportunity to progress toward theoretical perfection by identifying flaws to be avoided and best practices to be modeled in future studies. As Wallwork states, "Postmodernism helps investigators become aware of this situation and even more importantly, take moral responsibility for hidden biases and uses of power and knowledge."[20]

Key Positions in Multinational Research

Ruth Macklin's article, "Appropriate Ethical Standards" struck on many of the thoughts I have had surrounding research among minority or vulnerable communities, but in a multinational context. I agree with Macklin's assertion that people involved in research agree that the research "must adhere to appropriate ethical standards," but there is no concurrence of opinion about how to interpret and apply the concepts of ethical standards.[21] The seemingly overwhelming number of vagaries that permeate the discussion include questions about the nature of the standards, the people who should determine the standards, the universal applicability of the standards, and who ought to resolve disagreements about the standards and application in a multinational environment. All of these questions highlight the breadth and depth of the uncertainty that trouble the ethics of multinational human research projects.

Macklin goes on to discuss what she calls "ethical relativism" which she describes as variability of research rules and their application.[22] This is based on "the cultural norms accepted in the country in which the research is carried out" and the "economic disparity between industrialized countries and resource poor countries."[23] This directly impacts the type of research that can and ought to be considered in various countries be-

---

20 Ibid, p. 77.

21 Macklin, R. (2008). Models of institutional review board function. Emanuel, E. J., Grady, C., Crouch, R., Reidar, L., Miller, F., & Wendler, D. (Eds.). *The Oxford textbook of clinical research ethics*. New York, NY: Oxford University Press., p. 711.

22 Ibid, p. 712.

23 Ibid.

cause the standard of care based on the economic wealth of a region can and ought to determine what is an ethically acceptable treatment option. This is especially true if the research is funded by the economically disadvantaged country with no support or sponsor from a more economically prosperous region. Forcing researchers in developing countries to adhere to regulations developed by and for industrial countries could very easily be seen as ethical research jingoism. The flip side of that is the Pandora's Box that would be opened if researchers in poorer countries could ignore ethical standards set in wealthier countries. That might cause ethical relativism which would allow researchers to adopt any standard a country desired.

This leads to multitudinous views of whether an IRB from the sponsoring country, a research ethics committee from the developing country, or some variation of the two should review and approve the research project. An NBAC study suggests that the majority of both U.S. and developing country researchers believe that researchers should use international guidelines instead of U.S. regulations to cover joint projects. However, the use of international ethical codes and guidelines cannot address all the possible variations that might come up in the design and conduct of multinational research. There will necessarily be debate and negotiation among the groups involved in the research projects. While it may be difficult to establish an absolute standard or rule for multinational research, the goal of the review and approval process should be resolution of any differences with acknowledgement that everyone involved has the highest ethical standards in mind.

Barbara Koenig firmly believes that consent for a research study in its truest form should be about governance schemes based on deliberative theory which returns the consent concept to its original meaning in political philosophy and study participants giving "consent to be governed."[24] Koenig posits that individual autonomy is maintained even though control is given up with the study participant agreeing to accept someone else's idea of the best procedures and practices. This is summed up by Koenig's theory that a switch of focus from assessment of discrete data points to general governance is actually an example of personal sovereignty because "research participants who will share in the benefits of genomics knowledge are given the opportunity to consent to be governed."[25]

In general, I agree with this concept because the uncertainty and sheer potential volume of incidental results is outside of the basic idea of individual consent to participate in a study. Also, Koenig points out the obvious fact that "genomic research is observational, not interventional" which means most of the information gathered will be applicable on a population basis rather than an individual basis for a whole genome study.[26] That fact would not be valid for a narrow genetic test that is performed to assess a specific disease. The governance model is better suited to handle population level data and to maintain an ongoing relationship with the community as a whole whereas individual (participant by participant) processing of discrete, incidental data would be much harder to manage.

Additionally, an informed consent document could not comprehensively address all the possible variations of incidental findings during whole genomic research. Issues surrounding incidental findings remain, and range from clinical interpretation of data to utility in patient treatment and, more to the point for this specific topic, ethical obligations to return incidental findings that may arise from sequencing an entire

---

24 Koenig, B. A. (2014). Have we asked too much of consent? *The Hastings Center Report, 44*(4), 34. doi:10.1002/hast.329

25 Ibid.

26 Ibid.

genome. Effectively translating large amounts of genomic data into a concise report that physicians can accurately interpret and convey to patients is challenging. Many of the data found during whole genome analysis are of unknown significance and may or may not be causative.

There is also the dilemma of what to do with incidental findings if there is no treatment for a condition detected. Should those incidental findings be revealed? Is there an obligation to disclose findings from a child's genome study that do not currently pose a risk but which may manifest in adulthood, especially since the child being tested cannot consent? As with a great many topics in the ethics of research, there are a great many unresolved questions.

I understand skepticism about the composition of the CAB as proposed by Barbara Koenig. However, after doing a little checking into the source and nature of the CAB mentioned by Koenig, the intent and characteristics of the CAB seem to be ethically based. The CAB referenced by Koenig was an eventual iteration of a 4-day Deliberative Community Engagement Project (DCE) performed by the Mayo Clinic Biobank in September of 2007.[27] According to Olsen, "the DCE was designed to allow citizen input into biobank design and to assure that community values were taken into account. To achieve diverse perspectives, we selected twenty lay members of the Olmsted County, Minnesota community who varied by age, sex, social and economic status, race, ethnicity, and employment."[28] The DCE community members were given background information about biobanking issues. They then participated in a DCE event where they were able to listen to presentations and Q&A sessions with patient advocates, potential biobank researchers, experts on

27 Olson, J. E., Ryu, E., Johnson, K. J., Koenig, B. A., Maschke, K. J., Morrisette, J. A., … Cerhan, J. R. (2013). The Mayo Clinic Biobank: A building block for individualized medicine. Mayo Clinic Proceedings, 88(9), 952–962. http://doi.org/10.1016/j.mayocp.2013.06.006

28 Ibid.

biobanking procedures, human subjects, protection staff, and privacy experts.[29] Following the meetings, the community members made recommendations about biobank procedures and suggested guiding principles, including: the need for strong privacy protections, convenient recruitment, the importance of data sharing, limited options for return of research results, the importance of long-term community oversight, and an easy-to-understand consent document.[30] Following the DCE project about half of the community members later became standing members of the ongoing CAB at the Mayo Clinic Biobank. Supplemented by additional members, the CAB provides advice on management and operation of the Biobank, reviews policies, evaluates participant materials, and provides input on complex policy decisions such as data sharing and return of research results. The CAB meets quarterly, and has twenty members, and is co-chaired by a community member.[31] While there will probably always be situations where skepticism is warranted, sometimes we need to have faith that people are executing their duties with positive intent even if the outcome is less than ideal.

References

Emanuel, E. J., Grady, C., Crouch, R., Reidar, L., Miller, F., & Wendler, D. (Eds.). (2008). The Oxford textbook of clinical research ethics. New York, NY: Oxford University Press.

The Belmont Report. Retrieved from http://www.hhs.gov/ohrp/humansubjects/ guidance/belmont.html

---

29 Ibid, p. 954.

30 Ibid.

31 Ibid, p. 955.

Human Subjects Research. Code of Federal Regulations. (45 C.F.R. 46). (2009). Retrieved from http://www.hhs.gov/ohrp/humansubjects/guidance/45cfr46.html

Wertheimer, A. (2011) Rethinking the ethics of clinical research. New York, NY: Oxford University Press

The Belmont Report. Retrieved from http://www.hhs.gov/ohrp/humansubjects/guidance/belmont.html

NBAC. National Bioethics Advisory Commission. 2001. Ethical Policy Issues in International Research: Clinical Trials in Developing Countries. Volume 1: Report and Recommendations of the National Bioethics Advisory Commission. Bethesda, MD: NBAC. Available at http://bioethics.georgetown.edu/nbac/pubs.html

Joffe, S. & Truong, R. (2008). The ethics of placebo-controlled trials. In Emanuel, E. J., Grady, C., Crouch, R., Reidar, L., Miller, F., & Wendler, D. (Eds.). The Oxford textbook of clinical research ethics. (pp. 245-260). New York, NY: Oxford University Press.

Miller, F. (2008). Equipoise and randomization. In Emanuel, E. J., Grady, C., Crouch, R., Reidar, L., Miller, F., & Wendler, D. (Eds.). The Oxford textbook of clinical research ethics. (pp. 261-272). New York, NY: Oxford University Press.

Wallwork, E. (2008). Ethical analysis of research partnerships with communities. Kennedy Institute of Ethics Journal, 18(1), 57-85.

Fleischman, A.R. & Collogan, L.K. (2011). Research with children. Emanuel, E. J., Grady, C., Crouch, R., Reidar, L., Miller, F., & Wendler, D. (Eds.). The Oxford textbook of clinical research ethics. New York, NY: Oxford University Press.

Human Subjects Research. Code of Federal Regulations. (21 C.F.R. 53-4). (2009). Retrieved from http://www.hhs.gov/ohrp/humansubjects/guidance/21cfr53.html

Human Subjects Research. Code of Federal Regulations. (45 C.F.R. 46-7). (2009). Retrieved from http://www.hhs.gov/ohrp/humansubjects/guidance/45cfr46.html

Bowen, A. J. (2011). Models of institutional review board function. Emanuel, E. J., Grady, C., Crouch, R., Reidar, L., Miller, F., & Wendler, D. (Eds.). The

Oxford textbook of clinical research ethics. New York, NY: Oxford University Press.

http://www.fda.gov/RegulatoryInformation/Guidances/ucm126420.htm

http://www.hhs.gov/ohrp/archive/irb/irb_chapter1.htm

Macklin, R.. (2008). How Independent Are IRBs?. IRB: Ethics & Human Research, 30(3), 15–19. Retrieved from http://www.jstor.org.cuhsl.creighton.edu/stable/30033260

National Bioethics Advisory Commission. (2001). Ethical and Policy Issues in Research Involving Human Participants. Bethesda, Md.: National Bioethics Advisory Commission. Bethesda, MD: NBAC. http://bioethics.georgetown.edu/nbac/pubs.html

Wallwork, E. (2008). Ethical analysis of research partnerships with communities. Kennedy Institute of Ethics Journal, 18(1), 57-85.

Koenig, B. A. (2014). Have we asked too much of consent? The Hastings Center Report, 44(4), 33-34. doi:10.1002/hast.329

Macklin, R. (2008). Models of institutional review board function. Emanuel, E. J., Grady, C., Crouch, R., Reidar, L., Miller, F., & Wendler, D. (Eds.). The Oxford textbook of clinical research ethics. New York, NY: Oxford University Press.

National Bioethics Advisory Commission. (2001). Ethical and Policy Issues in International Research. Washington, D.C.: NBAC. Retrieved from http//:www.georgetown.edu/research/nrcbl/nbac/clinical/V011.pdf.

Olson, J. E., Ryu, E., Johnson, K. J., Koenig, B. A., Maschke, K. J., Morrisette, J. A., ... Cerhan, J. R. (2013). The Mayo Clinic Biobank: A building block for individualized medicine. Mayo Clinic Proceedings, 88(9), 952–962. http://doi.org/10.1016/j.mayocp.2013.06.006

Essay 6

PARADIGMS OF COMMUNITY PARTNERSHIP RESEARCH: APPLICATION AND SPECIFICATION, EXTENSION, AND POSTMODERN

Ernest Wallwork, in his article "Ethical Analysis of Research Partnerships with Communities," attempts to "identify the main ways of thinking ethically about the obligations of investigators and the roles and rights of communities in scientific research" through a review of the ever-growing literature on the subject.[32] In the analysis, Wallwork purports that the "advocates of community-partnership research implicitly adopt one of three models or paradigms for thinking ethically: application/specification; extension; and postmodern."[33] Within each of these three models, Wallwork highlights the key discussion points, pros and cons, and principles for applying the model to research. Quite often, this analysis requires a comparison to research ethics when applied to research among individuals with the standard usually being The Belmont Report and the Common Rule. While Wallwork's article gives a balanced presentation of each of the paradigms, I believe the extension model as it applies to community-based research has the best balance between protection if the individual and the community while being the most practically applicable of the paradigms. Therefore, the extension model is the preferred paradigm because it has the best balance between theory and practice.

The first model that Wallwork addresses is the application and speci-

---

32 Wallwork, E. (2008). Ethical analysis of research partnerships with communities. *Kennedy Institute of Ethics Journal, 18*(1), 57.

33 Ibid, p. 62.

fication model. This is so named because Wallwork views the model as the application and specification of the "current, individualistically oriented bioethics research guidelines, as articulated in documents like the Belmont Report and the Common Rule."[34] This model prioritizes the interests and autonomy of the individual over those of the larger community. In fact, the community's interests are important only in terms of the impact on the individual. Wallwork highlights quite clearly that the application and specification model is grossly inadequate ethically as a viable paradigm for community-based research when he explains that the "model rests on the liberal ideal of treating individuals as autonomous rational agents, conceived as unencumbered by communities, shared traditions, narratives, customs, values, and practices."[35] The idea that a study participant in a community-based research project can be separated from the greater community from which the participant derives her "identi[ty] and whose values, beliefs, and practices [she] internalizes" is bereft of the requisite ethical and moral grounding to be considered a viable paradigm.[36]

On the other extreme of the paradigm gradient is the postmodern model. In the postmodern model, the community's values, beliefs, and practices are given as much weight, if not more weight, than the autonomy of the individual. Postmodern concepts are starting to be addressed by the research community with the discussion focusing on community-research partnerships. Barbara Israel, Professor in the Department of Health Behavior and Health Education at the University of Michigan, has been widely published on topics related to conducting community-based participatory research in collaboration with partners in diverse ethnic

---

34 Ibid.

35 Ibid, p. 65.

36 Ibid.

communities. Israel supports the belief that researchers must take into account the import of "local knowledge" and combine that with "universal ethical principles and objective scientific truths."[37] Trying to inculcate the value, culture, tradition and history into community-based research can be a challenge. The gap between theory and practical application is both wide and deep. How does one assess if the IRB is adequately ascertaining the wants and needs of the community, or how does one determine if the IRB is paying due respect to the myths, customs, traditions, and values of the communities in which the research is being conducted? Moreover, who will select the person or people that will be responsible for judging the extent to which the IRB has attained a completely subjective standard of community consideration? At the end of the day, one needs to acknowledge that the process of conducting community-based research can never reach a point of absolute theoretical perfection. Rather, one must consider each community-based study as an opportunity to progress toward theoretical perfection by identifying flaws to be avoided and best practices to be modeled in future studies. As Wallwork states, "Postmodernism helps investigators become aware of this situation and even more importantly, take moral responsibility for hidden biases and uses of power and knowledge."[38]

The final paradigm for thinking ethically about community-partnership research discussed by Wallwork is the extension model which "takes up the issue of community respect in ways that go beyond the liberal individualism embedded in the application and specification model."[39] The

---

37 Israel, Barbara A.; Schulz, Amy J.; Parker, Edith A.; and Becker, Adam B. (1998). Review of Community-Based Research: Assessing Partnership Approaches to Improve Public Health. *Annual Review of Public Health* 19: 173–202.

38 Wallwork, E. (2008). Ethical analysis of research partnerships with communities. *Kennedy Institute of Ethics Journal, 18*(1), 77.

39 Ibid, p. 66.

extension model applies the individual concepts of harm, informed consent, and justice that are basic to The Belmont Report and the Common Rule to larger communities and group entities. Wallwork points out that the Belmont Report mandates the protection of "vulnerable populations from exploitation and other forms of injustice" which is often copied by researchers and applied to community-based research.[40] One might say that when the Belmont Report considers vulnerable populations such as welfare workers and prisoners, it does not give thought to the entire community. However, the extension model extends the protection and consideration of the individual to the larger community such as the Navajo who have distinctive ethnic features and histories and need to be treated with those factors in mind.

Wallwork breaks down the extension model into subsections including group harms, respect for community, group consent, and social justice. The extension model's application to the community is elucidated in the discussion about group harms and the "duty to minimize harm to research subjects gives rise to the obligation of investigators to try to protect the entire community from harms that go beyond the interests of the individual research subjects who are drawn from that community."[41] The most important part of group harm in the extension model is that the majority of the individuals in a group suffer harm because of "their identification with or participation in the group. Research that weakens shared beliefs, myths, rituals, institutions, practices, or identification with a group diminishes every member by virtue of the damage to the shared social structure and to the affective and cultural ties that bind the group together."[42]

---

40 Ibid, p. 71.

41 Ibid, p. 66.

42 Ibid, p. 67.

The sub-category of "respect for the community" further underscores the extension model's application of individual rights and protections to the greater community. Wallwork posits that "researchers must work to understand a group's beliefs, traditions, and practices relevant to the study, including unique cultural meanings, such as the sacredness of body parts and proper ways of disposing of them."[43] This seems like a basic concept, but might be easily overlooked in the formulation of community-based research study. Formalizing the concept into a paradigm like the extension model gives researchers something to use as a reference when developing researcher-community partnerships.

The idea of group consent is an extension of the idea of informed consent for individual research subjects to the larger community. This clearly supplants the autonomy of the individual with the importance of the community.[44] Wallwork considers "the key point [to be] that researchers need to take cognizance of existing inequalities and address them to some extent at the outset of a proposed study by negotiating benefits to an impoverished community in the context of a collaboration that is procedurally and substantively fair to both parties."[45] This provides a third solid support to the extension model so that it is a viable, ethical paradigm for community-based research.

The final aspect of the extension model is social justice. In social justice, the research-partnerships try to balance out the relationship between the researchers and the community so that the research practices are fairer and the community receives a direct benefit from the research study. Wallwork notes that the researchers should "also seek to improve social, health, and economic conditions in the developing world and strengthen

---

43 Wallwork, E. (2008). Ethical analysis of research partnerships with communities. *Kennedy Institute of Ethics Journal, 18*(1), 68.

44 Ibid.

45 Ibid, p. 69.

institutional structures in these comparatively weak communities."[46] This is the final piece that completes the extension model and serves to make it the most ethically and practically viable of the paradigms presented by Wallwork.

The extension model for community-based research is ethically and practically the preferred paradigm to use. The other two models are either too focused on the individual over groups (application and specification) or too hard to apply because of their lack of structure and clarity of application (postmodern). Some might suggest that postmodern is the superior model to use in the community research environment because of the heightened emphasis and sensitivity to community involvement in every step of the research including reviewing, conducting, and publishing. However, the extension model also pays due attention to the impact and effect on the community of the study and vice versa while also having a more streamlined and applicable study review and conduction process. Theories and ivory tower thinking are wonderful, but what really matters is real world application and the extension model has the best combination of both.

References

The Belmont Report. Retrieved from http://www.hhs.gov/ohrp/humansubjects/guidance/belmont.html

Israel, B. A., Krieger, J., Vlahov, D., Ciske, S., Foley, Mary, Fortin, P., ... Tang, G. (2006).

Challenges and Facilitating Factors in Sustaining Community-Based Partic-

---

46 Ibid, p. 70.

ipatory Research Partnerships: Lessons Learned from the Detroit, New York City and Seattle Urban Research Centers. Journal of Urban Health : Bulletin of the New York Academy of Medicine, 83(6), 1022–1040. http://doi.org/10.1007/s11524-006-9110-1

Israel, Barbara A.; Schulz, Amy J.; Parker, Edith A.; and Becker, Adam B. (1998). Review of Community-Based Research: Assessing Partnership Approaches to Improve Public Health. Annual Review of Public Health 19: 173–202.

NBAC. National Bioethics Advisory Commission. (2001). Ethical Policy Issues in International Research: Clinical Trials in Developing Countries. Volume 1: Report and Recommendations of the National Bioethics Advisory Commission. Bethesda, MD: NBAC. Retrieved from http://bioethics.georgetown.edu/nbac/pubs.html

Wallwork, E. (2008). Ethical analysis of research partnerships with communities. Kennedy Institute of Ethics Journal, 18(1), 57-85.

Essay 7

ETHICS OF COGNITIVE ENHANCEMENTS: COMPARISON OF VIEWS ON BENEFICENCE AND JUSTICE

Cognitive enhancement may be thought of as the amplification or extension of core capacities of the mind through improvement or augmentation of internal or external information processing systems. Cognitive enhancements can range from education, mental techniques, external technological devices, pharmacological products, mechanical, and genetic manipulations. While cognitive enhancement encompasses all of these means, the latter methods are more controversial and likely to provoke ethical concerns. Pharmacological cognitive enhancement involves the use of drugs and chemicals to improve cognitive function. Mechanical cognitive enhancement involves the integration of technology and the brain with devices like cochlear implants and hippocampal memory mediation chips or internal direct brain interfaces such as deep brain stimulation, and external direct brain interfaces such as electroencephalogram (EEG) electrode arrays. Genetic cognitive enhancement occurs when genes involved in any of the cognitive processes are manipulated through implantation of fetal neural tissue or stem cells differentiated into neural cells.

Presidential Commission

The Presidential Commission for the Study of Bioethical Issues published a study titled "Gray Matters Topics at the Intersection of Neuroscience, Ethics, and Society" that among other topics considers the ethics of cognitive enhancement. The Presidential Commission posits that "[m]odifying the brain and nervous system is not inherently ethically problematic."[47] They hold that people generally employ a wide array of modalities to modify the brain and nervous system including high-quality nutrition, meditation, education, drugs, and devices. The Presidential Commission covered the four principles of bioethics with one of the foci being the principle of beneficence and non-maleficence. This requires ensuring the wellbeing and health of those involved in the research while avoiding doing any harm. Ethically, we as a society have a responsibility to consider the potential benefits and risks of cognitive enhancements. Generally, most people would agree that anytime one can safely and effectively modify a person's neural network in order to achieve reduction of suffering and impairment then the steps taken are ethically acceptable.

---

47 Presidential Commission for the Study of Bioethical Issues. (2015). Capacity and the Consent, p. 40.

In fact, the Presidential Commission goes so far as to say that the "development and use of neural modifiers to maintain or improve health or treat disease represents one of the primary goals of neuroscience research and advances both individual and public beneficence."[48] Those cognitive enhancements may be beneficial to people suffering from diseases such as Parkinson's, Alzheimer's, and Huntington's even if the benefit does not extend to everyone in the society. Some interventions that would be universally seen as completely ethical would be taking a dietary supplement known to be safe or a prescription medication shown to be safe and effective by adequate scientific research to maintain or improve health or treat a disease or disorder. Cognitive enhancements that improve mental performance can also create significant instrumental benefits to both the individual and society. An individual may enjoy increased success at work, earning potential, greater chance of having social and economic success, and better overall health. Some of those benefits may be conferred on the society as a whole. Some cognitive enhancement modalities like education or those that treat or prevent disease, could be morally required in societies capable of delivering them because of their potential to advance both individual and public beneficence.

The bioethics principle of justice plays a role in the research and application of cognitive enhancement modalities. The Presidential Commission looked at justice from the perspective of an individual with enhanced cognitive abilities who might have an advantage relative to others which would make the enhancement a positional good because it gives an advantage to people who have it versus people who do not.[49] Social justice and fairness as it applies to cognitive enhancement does not only require

---

48 Ibid, p. 41.

49 Presidential Commission for the Study of Bioethical Issues. (2015). Capacity and the Consent.

that the benefit be equally distributed among society, but it also requires that the risk not be unduly placed on a single, vulnerable sector of society. Cognitive enhancement modalities can also confer non-positional benefits such as knowledge which is considered a good and holds inherent value. In this case, justice would be providing safe and efficacious cognitive enhancers that "can provide individuals with a greater range of opportunities and enabling them to participate more fully in society."[50] The Presidential Commission went on state that "The non-positional individual and societal benefits of neural modification support pursuing modifications collectively, rather than limiting access to a privileged few."[51] In some circumstances, cognitive enhancement interventions could be used to reduce inequities between the cognitively advantaged and disadvantaged. Some scholars argue that if cognitive enhancement and other neural modifiers could reduce existing educational performance inequities, then justice requires they be distributed across society.[52] Social justice and fairness require that inequities are minimized across society while beneficence is not given to a select entitled few and the risk burden is not carried by a vulnerable few, but rather both are equally distributed.

Bostrom and Sandberg

In their paper on cognitive enhancements, Bostrom and Sandberg cover much of the same ground as the Presidential Commission.[53] After

---

50 Ibid, p. 43.

51 Ibid, p. 44.

52 Sandberg, A., & Savulescu, J. (2011). The social and economic impacts of cognitive enhancement. In J. Savulescu, R. ter Meulen, and G. Kahane (Eds.). Enhancing Human Capacities. Malden, MA: Wiley-Blackwell.

53 Bostrom, N., & Sandberg, A. (2009). Cognitive Enhancement: Methods, Ethics, Regulatory.

covering the basics of what cognitive enhancemen is and which modalities function in which ways, Bostrom and Sandberg start to cover the ethics of cognitive enhancements. In terms of beneficence, they discuss the individual benefits of each treatment modality, but do not go into much depth as to the societal beneficence. They point out that education has many benefits beyond higher job status and salary such as reduced risk of substance abuse, crime and many illnesses while improving quality of life, social connectedness, and political participation. The authors go into more detail about the safety or non-maleficence of cognitive enhancements. Their consensus is that patient autonomy overrides at least minor medical risks even when the procedure does not reduce or prevent morbidity. Particularly in the case of medical cognitive enhancements, the user must be allowed to decide whether the benefits outweigh the potential risks, based on advice from medical professionals and her own estimates of how the intervention might affect her personal goals and her way of life.

Bostrom and Sandberg spend some time discussing the concepts of positional versus non-positional good and how it affects the ethics of cognitive enhancement. They believe that if cognitive enhancements were purely positional goods, then the pursuit of such enhancements would be a waste of time, effort, and money.[54] In effect, one person's gain would produce an offsetting negative externality of equal magnitude, resulting in no net gain in social utility to compensate for the costs of the enhancement efforts. They also posit that cognitive enhancements are also intrinsically desirable because the immediate value to the possessor does not entirely depend on other people lacking them. Having a good memory or a creative mind is normally valuable in its own right, whether or not other

---

54 Bostrom, N., & Sandberg, A. (2009). Cognitive Enhancement: Methods, Ethics, Regulatory Challenges. *Science & Engineering Ethics*, *15*(3), 311-341. doi:10.1007/s11948-009-9142-5

people also possess similar excellences. Furthermore, many cognitive capacities also have instrumental value, both for individuals and for society. Bostrom and Sandberg conclude that an enhancement that enables an individual to solve some of society's problems would produce a positive externality which would not only convey benefits for the enhanced individual, but the benefits would also carry over to other members of society.

Bostrom and Sandberg also consider the bioethics principle of justice in their discussion, but call it inequality.[55] They feel that cognitive enhancements might exacerbate social inequality by adding to the advantages of elites. To assess this concern one would have to consider whether future cognitive enhancements would be expensive or inexpensive and would also have to take into account that there is more than one dimension to inequality. Another dimension of inequality would be the gap between the cognitively gifted and the cognitively deficient. One should also have to consider under what conditions society might have an obligation to ensure universal access to interventions that improve cognitive performance. Bostrom and Sandberg look at public policy and regulations as the driving force "to either contribute to inequality by driving up prices, limiting access, and creating black markets; or reduce inequality by supporting broad development, competition, public understanding, and perhaps subsidized access for disadvantaged groups."[56]

Conclusion

While the paper from the Presidential Commission and the paper written by Bostrom and Sandberg use slightly different terminology and take slightly different tacks in their discussions, their conclusions on benefi-

---

55 Ibid.

56 Ibid, p. 329.

cence and justice are similar, as described in this paper. In fact, the high degree of concurrence between the two opinions on beneficence and justice is really only separated because Bostrom and Sandberg go into detail about the public policy and regulation that should accompany and enforce the bioethics principles that surround cognitive enhancements. Moving forward with cognitive enhancements seems inevitable and because these developments are happening in so many areas, case-by-case monitoring is necessary. However, because the developments are incremental, review and assessment of their effects is possible with regulations and policies put in place to manage the process.

References

Bostrom, N., & Sandberg, A. (2009). Cognitive Enhancement: Methods, Ethics, Regulatory

Challenges. Science & Engineering Ethics, 15(3), 311-341. doi:10.1007/s11948-009-9142-5

Harris, J. (2007). Enhancing Evolution: The Ethical Case for Making Better People. Princeton, NJ: Princeton University Press

Presidential Commission for the Study of Bioethical Issues. (2015). Capacity and the Consent Process. (Chapter 3, pp. 53-82) Gray matters: Topics at the intersection of neuroscience, ethics, and society. Vol 2. Retrieved from http://bioethics.gov/sites/default/files/GrayMatter_V2_508.pdf

Sandberg, A., & Savulescu, J. (2011). The social and economic impacts of cognitive enhancement. In J. Savulescu, R. ter Meulen, and G. Kahane (Eds.). Enhancing Human Capacities. Malden, MA: Wiley-Blackwell

Savulescu, J. (2006). Justice, fairness, and enhancement. Annals of the New York Academy of Science, 1093, 321-338; Buchanan, A. (2011). Better than Human: The Promise and Perils of Enhancing Ourselves (Philosophy in Action). New York, NY: Oxford University Press.

Case Study

Sam had been driving his SUV when his car skidded on ice as he crossed the bridge around the corner from his apartment. The car tumbled over the guardrail and landed in the icy river below, causing Sam to lose consciousness. The first responders estimated that Sam had spent at least ten minutes underwater before two civilians were able to remove him from the car and pull him to the riverbank. The civilians immediately began CPR, but Sam never regained consciousness after the incident.

Sam's parents refused to give up hope and decided to send him to a rehabilitation center. One day while searching online for studies on persistent vegetative state (PVS) patients, Sam's mother came across a study that examined new ways to communicate with patients. The researchers had discovered that some PVS patients were actually in a minimally conscious state (MCS) and could communicate with the researchers with the right technology.

Molly was a bright neurology resident who had decided to take a research year while preparing her application for a fellowship. She had chosen to work on the MCS project after seeing families struggle with end-of-life decisions for PVS and brain-dead patients. When she witnessed her mentor use the team's technology to interact with a patient who had been considered to be in PVS for the past five years, she was hooked.

Despite the breathtaking nature of their technology, however, the team members did not pretend to be miracle workers. They realized their technology was still in its infancy and would require thorough testing before it could be implemented across the country. Until then, use of the technology adhered to strict rules. It could only be used to elicit yes or no answers from the patients to questions that were limited to a specific list: Is the sky blue? Is the grass purple? The researchers did not want to ask anything serious that could potentially upset the study's participants.

Molly's mentor thought that Sam would be an ideal participant for the study. He had been a young healthy adult in his prime at the time of the accident, which had also occurred less than a year ago. The entire team was optimistic going into the testing session.

As Sam was wheeled into the testing room, his mother pulled Molly aside. "I know you're only supposed to ask him specific questions, but can you ask him if he wants all of this?" she asked. "Can you ask if he's in pain? Does he want us to keep providing care?"

Ethical Questions to Ponder

(1) Do we need to differentiate between patients who are in the vegetative versus the minimally conscious state when providing care to or withdrawing life support from them?

(2) Is it ethical for someone who cannot give consent to participate in research?

(3) Should participants with disorders of consciousness be enrolled in a clinical study?

Chapter 4

Philosophy:
Can Theory Meet Practice?

Throughout history, philosophers have tackled rather abstract questions. Mixed in among the subsets of philosophical thought such as metaphysics, ontology, epistemology, logic, and esthetics we find ethics which is primarily concerned with "the good."

One may conceive philosophical bioethics or medical ethics to be a critical evaluation of assumptions and arguments into norms, values, right and wrong, good and bad, what ought to be done and what ought to be left undone in the context of medical practice. On one hand, philosophical bioethics is simply an effort to create a framework by which to increase the rigor and thoughtfulness of medical decision-making. Building a defensible construct for medical practice based on universal principles to apply to any and all particular avenues of conduct in individual cases seems to be an unattainable goal. In the end, we may be best served to consider several competing theories based on widely accepted principles that we can attempt to apply to cases as we encounter them.

Discussion Topics

Infanticide

Theoretical ethics statement to evaluate and consider: "Anybody trying to justify the stoning as described in Jackson's "The Lottery" would have to assume a cultural relativist position, thus denying the relevance of ethics. However, the Groningen Protocol can be justified in terms of cultural diversity."

While Shirley Jackson intended "The Lottery" to be a commentary on American society's proclivity to blindly following traditions, one cannot help but see a similarity to the rituals practiced by the people of Pre-Colombian Mesoamerica and South America. The Maya, Inca, and Aztecs regularly sacrificed people, usually captured prisoners, but sometimes members of their own society (especially children), in order to control the weather and influence gods to favor them. The Lottery similarly sacrificed a member of their society in order to influence the harvest as Old Man Warner suggests when he says, "Lottery in June, corn be heavy soon." I mention this to bring back the idea that the argument supporting The Lottery is cultural relativism which holds that all cultural beliefs are equally valid and that truth itself is relative, depending on the cultural environment. Therefore, the entire situation of the Lottery might be morally bereft in modern Western ideology, but for the people who live in the fictitious society of The Lottery, all religious, ethical, esthetic, and political beliefs are completely relative to the individual within that specific society. One can say that the belief system and the sacrifice of the Lottery would not be ethical in one's own society and would be considered murder.

To compare the Lottery to the Groningen Protocol, the Groningen

Protocol is actually based on a modern, Western society and therefore we can better evaluate the ethics of the infanticide that their society permits. Some have suggested in this conversation that the euthanasia is permissible because it obviates the pain and suffering of the baby, the parents' emotional pain and suffering, and the future expense of raising the child to the point of natural mortality. Others have suggested that the entire idea is unethical because the child is a sentient being with the right of autonomy and self-determination. Also, not only is the information being used to make the determination suspect in quantity and quality, the parents' ability to weigh the information is dubious. Therefore, the decision to euthanize a particular infant is fraught with major ethical holes. Is cultural diversity enough to warrant this practice of infanticide? I do not think so because cultural diversity does not go as far as cultural relativism in terms of holding cultural beliefs to be equally valid or allowable.

Thomson's Violinist

Judith Jarvis Thomson's moral philosophy paper, "A Defense of Abortion," first published in 1971, is a collection of thought experiments centered on a violinist, an expanding child, and people-seeds. Thomson starts with the presupposition for the sake of argument that a fetus has a right to life, but argues that a fetus's right to life does not trump the pregnant woman's right to control her own body and life-support functions and, therefore, that induced abortion is not morally impermissible. While the pro-choice movement has held up Thomson's analogies as a brilliant discourse on abortion, many believe the analogies are a bit on the weak side and have received quite a bit of criticism from the pro-life movement over the years since 1971. While Thomson focuses her argument on the concept that the right to life does not guarantee the use of another's body against their will, there are other relevant factors that play a role in determining a person's rights in a given situation.

One can appreciate the fact that Thomson could not reasonably cover every single version of pregnancy in her discussion. For instance, none of Thomson's thought experiments covered consensual sex where no effort was made to prevent pregnancy. Thomson does discuss, and argues that abortion is acceptable in cases of pregnancy from rape (the Violinist experiment), pregnancy that threatens the mother's life (modified Violinist experiment and growing baby in the small house), and pregnancies where attempts were made to prevent the pregnancy (burglar and people seeds experiment). Thomson's arguments lose some strength because they are all predicated on the idea that the fetus has no rights (even though she pretends that she is considering the fetus a person) and the mother has rights that trump all others. She presents the argument as if this concept is a given when it is highly debatable. Also, her arguments lean to the illogical or fanciful side of things. One can hardly give credibility to an argument that stretches logic a little too much.

Analogical arguments have a place in moral reasoning and can provide some insight into the consistency of one's moral outlook. In order to construct a good analogical argument, the sub-argument for the analogy-stating premise needs to be strong and the evaluative premise must be more acceptable than the negation of the evaluative conclusion.[01] If the two premises are inadequate, then the opponents of the argument would reject the conclusion and, therefore, reject the evaluative premise.

Thomson's arguments are guided by some beliefs that deny moral relevance of several factors such as the difference between allowing a person to die versus murdering a person (a fetus) or the difference between using a house as a fetal incubator versus using a body to grow

---

01 Lo, N. (2004). *Analogical arguments*. Retrieved from http://philosophy.hku.hk/think/value/analogy.php (Links to an external site.)

a fetus.[02] These differences could be morally relevant which would then shift one's intuitive judgments about the imaginary scenarios and cause one to reject the application of the analogies to abortion.

Another aspect of Thomson's analogies that creates weakness is found in the "people seeds" analogy.[03] The whole idea of flying and nesting people seeds is fantastical and completely removed from reality as experienced by humans. Since Thomson's thought experiments attempt to elicit intuitions which are, in turn, reliant on our experience, one can justifiably reject the entire premise because the world Thomson presents is so bizarre and different from human reality. The difference between the "people seeds" scenario and reality is so dramatic that one cannot determine whether or not these seeds have rights and whether or not these rights outweigh our property rights. In essence, one can have no intuitive judgements about something so far beyond one's realm of experience, so the analogy fails.

Intention

Theoretical ethics statement to evaluate and consider: "There is a gray area in end-of-life care between treatments administered to relieve pain and suffering and those intended to shorten the dying process."

Charles Sprung, from the Department of Anesthesiology and Critical Care Medicine at Hadassah Medical Center in Israel, has written extensively about issues surrounding end-of-life decision-making. In one paper about the topic, the "gray area" mentioned by Sprung et al. is one of understanding of motive and intent rather than one of scientific under-

---

02 Thomson, J.J. (1971). A Defense of Abortion. *Philosophy & Public Affairs*, *1*(1), 47-66.
03 Ibid.

standing.[04] In other words, the physicians are not misunderstanding the dosing of medications, but rather they are conflicted about, or hesitant to fully disclose, the actual outcome being sought by a certain dosing regimen. Sprung et al. believe that the "[d]ifferentiation between the two is complicated and may be impossible because the physicians' true intentions are often difficult to ascertain...these intentions are likely to be multilayered, complex, and ambiguous."[05] Even self-reporting may not lend much clarity to the physicians' intent because the physicians may feel guilty about their intent and not want to admit to an action that others may find ethically questionable.

Another area that might contribute to "gray area" effect may also be attributed to the actual effect of the drug on the patient. While Sprung et al. found a correlation between the dosing of a drug and the patient's life expectancy when the explicit intent was euthanasia or SDP, one can not determine intent by analyzing the absolute dose of drugs.[06] In fact, the "prior exposure, tolerance, and duration of medications" may confound the determination of intent based on absolute dose because those factors will create varying effects on the patient.[07] This may contribute to the inadequate dosing of drugs for SDP or overdosing drugs for palliative care and pain management as much as a physician's fear of prosecution for SDP or a physician's unconsciously disguising SDP as palliative care.

This difference of opinion is mainly based on the idea of how teleology deals with the concept of the goal of life. According to the Encyclopedia Britannica, "Teleological theories differ on the nature of the end that ac-

---

04 Sprung, C.L. et al. (2008). Relieving suffering or intentionally hastening death: Where do you draw the line? *Critical Care Medicine*, *36*(1), 8-13.

05 Ibid, p. 11.

06 Sprung, C.L. et al. (2008). Relieving suffering or intentionally hastening death: Where do you draw the line? *Critical Care Medicine*, *36*(1), 8-13.

07 Ibid. 12.

tions ought to promote."[08] The Encyclopedia goes on to list subtypes including hedonism, universalistic hedonism, despotism, pragmatism, and existentialism which highlights the great range and scope of how people view the application of teleology.[09]

Consequently, instead of holding that SDP is counter to teleology based on death not being a goal of life, I posit teleology can be applied to individual time periods or instances in life. Since people naturally have different values as a result of the vast cultural diversity in the world, each individual must weigh the act of death against current suffering and confirm that they must know that death will relieve them of their current suffering. Therefore, an individual may find SDP or euthanasia to be their greatest good and the morally correct goal or end for that individual.

On the other hand, looking at SDP and euthanasia from a deontological perspective, and following Emmanuel Kant's teachings, euthanasia would be viewed as wrong. As deontology would argue, "the basic standards for an action's being morally right are independent of the good or evil generated."[10] The steps that are taken to end someone's life would be deemed medically unethical because the action would be counter to the physicians' ethical imperatives. The ideal deontological action would be to provide palliative care and ease the individual's pain and suffering as much as possible thereby allowing them to live their final days as comfortably as possible.

Free Will and "Mercy Killing"
Theoretical ethics question for evaluation and consideration: Is the act of "mercy" killing fully voluntary, or is a health professional

---

08 teleological ethics. (2016). In *Encyclopædia Britannica*. Retrieved fromhttp://www.britannica.com/topic/teleological-ethics

09 Ibid.

10 Ibid.

who engages in mercy killing somehow coerced by his/her emotions and hence not fully free?

Thomas Aquinas in Summa Theologiae theorized that human actions are those over which one has voluntary control and is a function of both intellect and will.[11] However, Aquinas pointed out that volition can be influenced by an emotion like fear (threat) or concupiscence (temptation), a force that Aquinas calls coercion.[12] One consequently wonders if the coercive effect carries over to other emotions or to extreme situations like the effect of compassion on health professionals engaged in "mercy killing" and if those circumstances cause the act to not be fully voluntary.

Because compassion is more similar in nature to concupiscence than to fear, compassion would serve to support or bolster one's will, thereby making one's actions voluntary. So, the "will" portion of voluntary action has been satisfied. On the other hand, Aquinas stresses that the pressure from temptation diminishes voluntariness because temptation affects the intellect (reason) and limits consideration of a possible act.[13] To be fully voluntary, an action would need to be wholly voluntary in both intellect and will.

Because compassion would serve to reinforce the professional's will, we are half way to considering the act voluntary. One may have the initial thought that compassion would lead a physician to impulsively go against training and immediately disregard palliative care in favor of euthanasia as the only possible solution to the patient's suffering. I believe that physicians would evaluate each option available to them for each patient and proceed until each option has been exhausted. If "mercy killing" is finally

---

11 Aquinas, T. (approx. 1270). Summa theologiae (IaIIae. Q6: The voluntary and the involuntary). Retrieved from http://www.newadvent.org/summa/2006.htm

12 Ibid.

13 Ibid.

decided upon, then it would be from both will and reason acting together. Opinions will vary throughout the medical community because of the natural variation in will, reason, and values among professionals, but I do not think compassion would make one act less than fully voluntarily in "mercy killing."

The fact that a health provider needs to worry or fear what a third party will think about the course of treatment is anathematic to the practice of medicine. Medicine was not intended to be practiced out of fear, but within the tenets of autonomy, beneficence, non-maleficence, and justice.

This is not to say that fear is completely absent in the mind of a healthcare professional. In fact, Danielle Ofri, an ED physician, wrote a book that deals with what a physician feels that speaks directly to fear in patient care. Ofri believes, and I concur, that fear is "a primal emotion in the practice of medicine."[14] The fear of making a mistake and causing harm never goes away, even with decades of experience, but it should be fear of violating non-maleficence not fear of what society or others will think.

Now, is this fear of violating non-maleficence coercive? I contend that this fear would steel one's will and strengthen one's conviction that one needs to do the utmost to best serve the patient's wellbeing. This fear might make one hesitate or question one's own decision in times of emergent, acute trauma, but hopefully only long enough to verify information and maybe confer with a colleague to confirm a treatment plan.

If fear of third party ramifications plays a role in patient care, then it might speak more to the nature of our society than the nature of the healthcare provider. My father and grandparents all practiced medicine and none of them mentioned fear of litigation or censure by a board of medicine as a concern during their careers. I am interested to hear my

---

14 Ofri, D. (2013). *What Doctors Feel: How Emotions Affect the Practice of Medicine*. Boston: Beacon Press.

fellow students' opinions about how fear has affected their approach to patient care.

Assisting in suicide and forgoing life-sustaining treatment
Theoretical ethics statement for evaluation and consideration:
"The anesthesiologist who finally withdrew Mr. Piergiorgio Welby's
ventilator (after administering sedatives to suppress the patient's
sense of dyspnea) assisted in the patient's suicide, if not from a legal
perspective then at least ethically."

The thesis implies that physician-assisted patient suicide is ethically worse than one might first consider withdrawing of life support to be. So, in this case, the suggestion is that the anesthesiologist's action was unethical because the action is being equated to an unethical action. I contend that the distinction between the withdrawal or withholding of life support and physician-assisted suicide or euthanasia as simply the difference between passive and active courses of action on the part of the physician and ethically not dissimilar from each other. That is not to say that the act is in and of itself unethical. Using Immanuel Kant's moral theory, which states that the rightness or wrongness of actions does not depend on the consequences but on whether they fulfill one's duty, will provide a helpful framework within which to consider the case of the anesthesiologist and Muscular Dystrophy patient.

According to Kant, moral worth only comes when one does something because of known duty regardless of whether one derived pleasure from the action.[15] From Kant's perspective, the anesthesiologist's decision to withdraw ventilator support would need to be evaluated according to whether one can create a maxim or universal law based on the action.

---

15 Kant, I. (1785). Groundwork for the Metaphysics of Morals. Retrieved from http://site.ebrary.com/lib/creighton/reader.action?docID=10170770

Maxims, and the universal laws that result from them, can be specified in a way that reflects all of the relevant features of the situation. Given the specificity of the situation, I posit that the anesthesiologist's action is not ethically dissimilar from physician-assisted patient suicide. This view is also held by James Rachels who argues that, "[i]f a doctor lets a patient die, for humane reasons, he is in the same moral position as if he had given the patient a lethal injection for humane reasons."[16] From a Kantian perspective, the physician fulfilled his duty by ending the suffering of the patient which would make the action ethical.

The difference in interpretation of both Kant's philosophy and the thesis query has made the discussion quite interesting. I still maintain that my original post was accurate in terms of Kant's meaning and the thesis. First, the thesis asked if the anesthesiologist's action was the same as assisted suicide. There was no mention of the general bioethical implications of the action therefore, beneficence, non-maleficence, autonomy, and justice are not part of this discussion (at least as related to the evaluation of the thesis), but may be relevant tangentially to the discussion. So, when one considers the thesis as just framed within the Kantian philosophy removing the ventilator in this specific situation is the same as assisted suicide.

Furthermore, the word "duty" in Kant's ethics does not mean social expectations, societal laws, group rules, professional guidelines, etc., but rather rationality or more specifically "what one would do if one were fully rational."[17] In fact, Robert Johnson of Stanford University contends

---

16 Rachels, J. (1986). Active and passive euthanasia. In J. Rachels, The end of life: Euthanasia and morality (99-122). New York, NY: Oxford University Press, p. 107.

17 Baron, M. (2002). Acting from duty. In A. Woods (Ed.), *Rethinking the Western Traditions: Groundwork for the Metaphysics of Morals*. (pp. 92-110). New Haven, CT, USA: Yale University Press. Retrieved from http://site.ebrary.com/lib/creighton/reader. action?docID=10170770 (Links to an external site.) p. 95.

that Kant argued, "we must act only as this fundamental law of (practical) reason prescribes, a law that would prescribe how any rational being in our circumstances should act."[18] This clearly means that the physician's medical ethics play no role in deciding if the action was within a universal law. Therefore, we may agree that rationality is what bestows dignity on human beings, and we must respect people's dignity. Therefore, a human being who may lose their dignity and their rationality through illness and pain may legitimately request euthanasia. We respect and protect their dignity by helping them die in circumstances of their own choosing.

This leads directly to my final point that Kant's second formulation which states that "we should never act in such a way that we treat Humanity, whether in ourselves or in others, as a means only but always as an end in itself."[19] Johnson goes on to explain that "[o]ur 'Humanity' is that collection of features that make us distinctively human, and these include capacities to engage in self-directed rational behavior and to adopt and pursue our own ends, and any other capacities necessarily connected with these."[20] I contend that the patient is not using the physician as a means to an end because the patient does not diminish the value of the physician as an individual in the relationship. However, if the physician would not have normally agreed to perform the procedure and the patient lied to the physician and tricked her into performing it, then the patient would have used the physician as a means to an end. This might be a situation where a patient wants to commit suicide and lies to a physician about the level of pain to obtain a large quantity of powerful narcotics, and then takes all the medicine at once and dies. Since the patient and physician maintained mutual respect for each other's

18 Johnson, R. (2014). Kant's Moral Philosophy. In E. Zalta (Ed.), *The Stanford Encyclopedia of Philosophy*. Retrieved from http://plato.stanford.edu/entries/kant-moral/

19 Ibid.

20 Ibid.

humanity, then there was no violation of Kant's second formulation.

The Utilitarian Calculus

Theoretical ethics statement for evaluation and consideration: "John Stuart Mill would agree with the authors of the Groningen Protocol that the Protocol is justified from a utilitarian perspective."

The Groningen Protocol was developed "for cases in which a decision is made to actively end the life of a newborn" in order to facilitate the legal assessment process and avoid potential police investigation.[21] While the Groningen Protocol does not settle the euthanasia debate, the specificity of Groningen Protocol provides a limited framework to focus the debate so fruitful discussion can proceed. We can further focus the discussion by considering the Protocol from the viewpoint of John Stuart Mill's classical utilitarianism.

We evaluate the Protocol by considering JS Mill's Utility Principle which states that "actions are right in proportion as they tend to promote happiness, wrong as they tend to produce the reverse of happiness."[22] When combined with Mill's statement that "[n]o person is an isolated being," then happiness is an aggregate happiness of everyone affected by the action which, in this situation, would include the infant, the parents, the physician and medical team, the friends and family of the infant and parents, and the community/society.[23]

Because the Protocol mandated that the infant have an independently

---

21 Verhagen, E., & Sauer, P.J.J. (2005). The Groningen Protocol-Euthanasia in Severely Ill Newborns. *New England Journal of Medicine*, *352*, 959-962.

22 Mill, J. S. (2011). On Liberty. Luton, Bedfordshire, GBR: AUK Classics. Retrieved from http://www.ebrary.com

23 Mill, J. S. (2011). On Liberty. Luton, Bedfordshire, GBR: AUK Classics. Retrieved from http://www.ebrary.com, p. 98.

confirmed diagnosis that includes "hopeless and unbearable suffering," one can readily see that the quantitative and qualitative aggregate happiness/pain balance would justify euthanasia.[24] The infant's pain and suffering would end immediately and the family/friends' emotional pain would increase in the short-term, but overall would be decreased because they would not need to see this child endure daily, unremitting suffering. Given that the happiness balance favors euthanasia and Ozolins' argument that "utilitarianism suggests that, for many people who are living lives of permanent suffering, their lives are not worth living," one can infer that JS Mill would have agreed with the Groningen Protocol.[25]

Principlism

If one were to start with ethical principlism based on the common ground moral principles of autonomy, beneficence, non-maleficence, and justice, then one can envision the framework for a practical approach for ethical decision-making. The practicality of this approach is that principlism is consistent with, or at the very least is not in conflict with, an array of ethical approaches towards moral decision-making. This point has received support from Ozolins—who posits that regardless of what the "starting point in moral theory might be—whether it is utilitarianism, virtue ethics, deontology or natural law—...the more likely we are to reach an agreed decision on a moral question."[26] Clearly, Ozolins views principlism as a structure within which one can apply moral theories to make decisions about specific clinical questions such as the patient with

---

24 Verhagen, E., & Sauer, P.J.J. (2005). The Groningen Protocol-Euthanasia in Severely Ill Newborns. *New England Journal of Medicine, 352,* 959-962.

25 Ozolins, J. (2015). Rationality in utilitarian thought. In Ozolins J.T. & Grainger, J. (Eds), *Foundations of healthcare ethics: Theory to practice* (pp. 102-119). Cambridge, UK: Cambridge Univ. Pr. p. 117.

26 Ibid, p. 33.

dementia who requires artificial nutrition and hydration, but constantly pulls out the tube due to fear and lack of understanding.

Several commentators, Ozolins and Smith Itlis among them, hold the belief that principlism allows for moral justification of an action rather than moral truth or rightness.[27] [28] Because the goal of bioethics is about case-resolution, one should focus on practical decision-making via the method that proves most fruitful. Analyzing a clinical situation by raising ethical questions within the framework of beneficence, non-maleficence, autonomy, and justice, clinicians can better elucidate how each question and answer fits the normative moral theories and produces a justifiable resolution. This means that principlism can indeed prove useful in analyzing the clinical situation posed in the posted question.

One can readily see the transient aspect of autonomy when one considers how other decisions one makes in life change depending on the season in which one finds oneself. The patient autonomously decided for nutrition and hydration support in her advanced directive (AD), but a person cannot possibly envision every potentiality that might arise in their future healthcare needs. In this case, we do not know what the patient understood in terms of informed consent prior to making her AD, but one could correctly determine that patient did not foresee that her dementia would cause her to be so afraid of the treatment that the only way to keep her from pulling out the line was to restrain her physically or chemically. One might validly argue the same point and posit that we review the degree of her ability in the current state to make decisions. I think that one should follow that review of the patient's autonomy with an evaluation of what steps should be executed next.

---

27 Ibid.

28 Smith Iltis, A. (2000) Bioethics as methodological case resolution: Specification, specified principlism and casuistry', *Journal of Medicine and Philosophy*, *25*(3), 271 - 284.

Ideally, the patient included provisions for a healthcare surrogate in her AD or Living Will and the medical team can get the surrogate to determine, through informed consent, what steps to take next. This is necessary because an attempt to maintain autonomy must be made even though "in practice the principle of beneficence—that is, to act in the patient's best interests—may be the dominant principle" in this situation.[29] Ozolins further argues that "certain patients cannot or do not know what is in their best interests...and that respect for autonomy should be overridden by the principle of beneficence."[30] This give-and-take among beneficence, nonmaleficence, autonomy, and justice in terms of prioritization in the decision-making process underlines the fact that the four principles function as a framework and not as strict, absolute moral laws.

Autonomy *vs* Vulnerability

Ralph McInerny's Ethica Thomistica is one of the widely recognized introductions to understanding the moral philosophy of St. Thomas Aquinas. In reading the book, one of the areas that really struck a chord with me was McInerny's comment that when taking "a course in ethics, we are given for analysis moral problems of an altogether too dramatic sort."[31] As McInerny points out, the implication of using such extreme moral dilemmas to test someone's ethics is that those questions suggest that we rarely encounter ethical dilemmas and may not encounter one in the future.[32] This is not the case for medical professionals because we are

---

29 Ozolins, J. (2015). Ethical principlism. In Ozolins J.T. & Grainger, J. (Eds), *Foundations of healthcare ethics: Theory to practice* (pp. 33-50). Cambridge, UK: Cambridge Univ. Pr. p. 58.

30 Ibid.

31 McInerny, R. (1997). *Ethica Thomistica*. Washington, DC: Catholic University of America Press. Chapters 6 and 7. p. 93.

32 Ibid.

confronted with practice ethics on a daily basis.

By practicing morally good and ethical medicine on a daily basis, we reinforce our character and decision-making which refines our concept of self. Our refined sense of "self" evaluates the situation and makes the decision or takes action based on all those daily character-defining moments in life up to that point. All those antecedent situations dealing with patients who are ill and, therefore, can be perceived as more vulnerable serve to form the framework within which we can make good moral decisions when faced with tough situations. However, the moral quality of the decision or action is determined by the moral quality of the life we live. As McInerny argues, "since human actions by definition proceed from reason and will, and are either good or bad, in order to be good they must proceed from correct reason and from a will that is oriented to the good."[33] If we do not make daily decisions or take action based in moral goodness, then we are highly unlikely to make good morally decisions in those moral outlying situations.

Vulnerability is essential for us to have a meaningful human connections as healthcare providers. By being vulnerable and having a will centered on moral goodness, we gain authenticity and sincerity which enable us to truly connect with our patients. Physicians need to partner with their patients, rather than simply treat disease. As Dr. William Osler, one of the founders of Johns Hopkins Hospital stated, "The good physician treats the disease; the great physician treats the patient who has the disease."[34] By connecting with the patient through the virtue of vulnerability, we will be able to achieve greater results in a patient's healthcare

---

33 McInerny, R. (1997). *Ethica Thomistica*. Washington, DC: Catholic University of America Press. Chapters 6 and 7. p. 95.

34 Centor, R. M. (2007). To Be a Great Physician, You Must Understand the Whole Story. *Medscape General Medicine*, 9(1), 59.

outcomes.

If those in the medical field were to be more vulnerable, embrace their emotions, and really connect with their patients, then the concern about developing special guidelines for dealing with vulnerable populations would be unnecessary. We would not need to worry about how vulnerable patients are treated because we would treat every patient like a vulnerable patient. The patient is a person, not a disease you are treating. It should be acceptable to shed a tear after giving a difficult diagnosis, hug a patient after a medical triumph, or speak to colleagues about how you are feeling after an emotionally draining day. Vulnerability is a virtue in medicine.

References

Jackson, S. (1948). The Lottery. The New Yorker. June 26, 1948.

Verhagen, E., & Sauer, P.J.J. (2005). The Groningen Protocol-Euthanasia in Severely Ill Newborns. New England Journal of Medicine, 352, 959-962.

Lo, N. (2004). Analogical arguments. Retrieved from http://philosophy.hku.hk/think/value/analogy.php (Links to an external site.)

Thomson, J.J. (1971). A Defense of Abortion. Philosophy & Public Affairs, 1(1), 47-66.

Miller, S. (2016). Week 3 discussion post in MHE605. Retrieved from: https://blueline.instructure.com/courses/1071203/discussion_topics/3168443?module_item_id=10446159

Sprung, C.L. et al. (2008). Relieving suffering or intentionally hastening death: Where do you draw the line? Critical Care Medicine, 36(1), 8-13.

teleological ethics. (2016). In Encyclopædia Britannica. Retrieved fromhttp://www.britannica.com/topic/teleological-ethics

Aquinas, T. (approx. 1270). Summa theologiae (IaIIae. Q6: The voluntary and the involuntary). Retrieved from http://www.newadvent.org/summa/2006.htm

Ofri, D. (2013). What Doctors Feel: How Emotions Affect the Practice of Medicine. Boston: Beacon Press.

Baron, M. (2002). Acting from duty. In A. Woods (Ed.), Rethinking the Western Traditions: Groundwork for the Metaphysics of Morals. (pp. 92-110). New Haven, CT, USA: Yale University Press. Retrieved from http://site.ebrary.com/lib/creighton/reader.action?docID=10170770 (Links to an external site.)

Johnson, R. (2014). Kant's Moral Philosophy. In E. Zalta (Ed.), The Stanford Encyclopedia of Philosophy. Retrieved from http://plato.stanford.edu/entries/kant-moral/

Kant, I. (1785). Groundwork for the Metaphysics of Morals. Retrieved from http://site.ebrary.com/lib/creighton/reader.action?docID=10170770 Rachels, J. (1986). Active and passive euthanasia. In J. Rachels, The end of life: Euthanasia and morality (99-122). New York, NY: Oxford University Press

Mill, J. S. (2011). On Liberty. Luton, Bedfordshire, GBR: AUK Classics. Retrieved from http://www.ebrary.com

Mill, J. S. (2001). Utilitarianism. London, GBR: ElecBook. Retrieved from http://www.ebrary.com

Ozolins, J. (2015). Rationality in utilitarian thought. In Ozolins J.T. & Grainger, J. (Eds), Foundations of healthcare ethics: Theory to practice (pp. 102-119). Cambridge, UK: Cambridge Univ. Pr.

Verhagen, E., & Sauer, P.J.J. (2005). The Groningen Protocol-Euthanasia in Severely Ill Newborns. New England Journal of Medicine, 352, 959-962.

Ozolins, J. (2015). Ethical principlism. In Ozolins J.T. & Grainger, J. (Eds), Foundations of healthcare ethics: Theory to practice (pp. 33-50). Cambridge, UK: Cambridge Univ. Pr.

Smith Iltis, A. (2000) Bioethics as methodological case resolution: Specification, specified principlism and casuistry', Journal of Medicine and Philosophy, 25(3), 271 - 284.

Centor, R. M. (2007). To Be a Great Physician, You Must Understand the Whole

Story. Medscape General Medicine, 9(1), 59.

McInerny, R. (1997). Ethica Thomistica. Washington, DC : Catholic University of
America Press. Chapters 6 and 7.

Essay 8

Do Not Resuscitate Order and Cardiopulmonary Resuscitation: A Utilitarian Perspective

Introduction

The arguments surrounding Do Not Resuscitate orders are not as
straight forward as one might conceive at first blush. When considering
the issue of to resuscitate or not to resuscitate, to borrow from Shakespeare's Hamlet, one must give equal weight to the status of both brain
and body after resuscitation or after death.[35] Hamlet asks the question for
all dejected souls—is it nobler to live miserably or to end one's sorrows
with a single stroke?[36] He knows that the answer would be undoubted-
ly "yes" if death were like a dreamless sleep devoid of tortuous nightmares,
but the "rub" or obstacle Hamlet faces is the fear that he does not know
what happens after death.[37] The same can be said for the use of Do Not

---

35 Shakespeare, W. & Froumentin, M. (2001). *The tragedy of Hamlet, Prince of Denmark*.
Retrieved from https://www.w3.org/People/maxf/XSLideMaker/hamlet.pdf

36 Ibid.

37 Ibid.

Resuscitate (DNR) orders and cardiopulmonary resuscitation (CPR) in the hospital setting. One must necessarily consider the relative physical and cognitive dysfunction to which a patient will be subjected if CPR is successful and the patient is brought back to life. Currently, the standard in hospitals is "always resuscitate unless there is a Do-Not-Resuscitate (DNR) order." This paper will use a classical utilitarian point of view to consider the argument for replacing the current rule with the rule to "never resuscitate unless there is a CPR order" for hospitalized patients.

Do Not Resuscitate Order—What, How, Why

A Do Not Resuscitate (DNR) order is a medical order written by a doctor after discussion with the patient or the patient's surrogates that instructs health care providers not to do cardiopulmonary resuscitation (CPR) if a patient suffers cardiac arrest or respiratory arrest. The DNR order is a prospective document in that the patient decides before an emergency occurs if CPR, intubation, defibrillation, etc. should be employed. The DNR order is specific to CPR, which includes rescue breathing to oxygenate the blood and chest compressions to circulate the blood through the body, but does not provide instructions to cease any other treatment, such as pain medicine, other medicines, or nutrition.[38] The ancillary treatments are only continued due to not being addressed in the DNR, not because the treatments are fundamentally important if a patient codes. This highlights the fact that the DNR has some major areas that are not given full consideration.

According to the American Medical Association (AMA) guidelines, consent to administer CPR is presumed since the patient is incapable of

---

38 Handley, A. (2001). Do not resuscitate. *Heart, 86*(1), 1–2. http://doi.org/10.1136/heart.86.1.1

communicating his or her treatment preference at the moment of arrest, and failure to act immediately is certain to result in the patient's death.[39] This presumption of automatically engaging in CPR has one definitive exception and one subjective exception. If the patient has an advanced directive or a DNR order to forgo CPR in the case of an emergency, then CPR must be withheld. CPR should also be withheld if there is no DNR order in place and the patient is incapable of expressing his or her desire, but the patient's family or surrogate medical decision maker prefer not to resuscitate. More subjectively, CPR may be withheld if, in the judgment of the treating physician, an attempt to resuscitate the patient would be futile. The AMA issued a set of guidelines to assist medical professionals and administrators in developing policies and procedures specific to such emergency situations.[40] The medical profession relies heavily on such guidelines to provide consistency across the healthcare industry, however, each health system has the autonomy to develop their own policy and procedures.

Some commentators, such as Anthony Handley, the past Chairman of the Resuscitation Council in Britain, insist that because CPR can be traumatic and invasive, performing CPR "when there is no reasonable hope of success is to deprive a human being of a dignified death."[41] Similarly, the default thought process of health systems and the AMA has been to encourage all patients to express in advance their preferences regarding the extent of treatment after cardiopulmonary arrest, especially patients at substantial risk of such an event. During discussions regarding patients' preferences, physicians should include a description of the

39 American Medical Association. (1991). Guidelines for the appropriate use of do-not resuscitate orders. *JAMA*.*265*(14):1868-1871. doi:10.1001/jama.1991.03460140096034.

40 American Medical Association. (1991). Guidelines for the appropriate use of do-not resuscitate orders. *JAMA*.*265*(14):1868-1871. doi:10.1001/jama.1991.03460140096034.

41 Handley, A. (2001). Do not resuscitate. *Heart*, *86*(1), 1–2. http://doi.org/10.1136/heart.86.1.1

procedures encompassed by CPR and the expected outcomes. Patients' preferences should be documented as early as possible and should be revisited and revised as appropriate.

The AMA has also provided guidelines for physicians if a patient or the patient's surrogate requests resuscitation that the physician determines would not be medically effective. In Opinion 2.037 on the "Medical Futility in End-of-Life-Care," the AMA recommends that "the physician should seek to resolve the conflict through a fair decision-making process, when time permits."[42] The consideration of patients' outcomes after CPR is an area that plays a significant role in determining the ethics of CPR and DNR.

CPR—Patient Outcomes

In the case of cardiopulmonary resuscitation, one must first determine how to define a successful outcome. While the immediate restoration of pulse would technically be necessary and sufficient to be a successful outcome, one should also consider survival to discharge, the quality of life, and the patient's physical, psychosocial, and emotional function. Uncertainty still exists about outcomes and many studies report 7 to 20% survivals to discharge depending on pre-hospital condition.[43] [44] The survival rate is dependent upon prior functioning and illness for institutionalized patients with those of poor functioning and chronic illness having the worst chance of survival. Among the frail and old,

42 Rien de Vos, Hanneke, de Haes, Koster and deHaan, (1999). Quality of survival after cardiopulmonary resuscitation. *Archives of Internal Medicine*. *159* pp. 249-254.

43 Cotler, M. (2000). Do Not Resuscitate Order; Clinical and Ethical Rationale and Implications, The *Medicine and Law* 19(3), 623-634.

44 Ehlenbach, W., Barnato, A., Curtis, J., Kreuter, W., Koepsell, T., Deyo, R., & Stapleton, R. (2009). Epidemiologic Study of In-Hospital Cardiopulmonary Resuscitation in the Elderly. New England Journal of Medicine 361:22-31. DOI: 10.1056/NEJMoa0810245

especially transfers from nursing homes to the hospital, survival is reported at less than 5% probability of leaving the hospital, and 0 to 4% survival at 180 days post-discharge.[45][46] These numbers are far lower than most patients probably believe the chances of recovery after CPR would be. Many patients would prefer to have CPR if the chance of a positive outcome is highly likely, but would prefer DNR if the outcome is likely to be negative.

Cotler also noted that clinicians are concerned with the level of pain suffered by patients resuscitated for a brief period of time only to die shortly thereafter.[47] This echoes the concerns of Handley and points to the fact that CPR is not a benign intervention, but rather an intervention with consequences for the patient aside from return to life. In a study of 827 patients in tertiary care facilities in Holland, 385 had immediate restoration of pulse and 162 survived to discharge, but five of those patients were in persistent coma. Of the patients who survived to discharge, fifty-one died after discharge with four deaths within three months and twenty-nine deaths within six months.[48] Rien De Vos et al. also found that patients who were comatose or had a stroke had the poorest outcome after CPR. This is a factor that healthcare system ethicists should consider when developing DNR order informed consent processes.

The quality of life after successful resuscitation is to a large extent influenced by the post-CPR neurological condition of the patient. A number of neurological disorders occur after CPR in approximately one-

45 Rozenbaum, E. & Shenkman, L. (1988). Predicting Outcomes of In-Hospital Cardiopulmonary Resuscitation. Critical Care Medicine.

46 Tomlinson T. & Brody, H. (1988). Ethics and communication in do not resuscitate orders. *New England Journal of Medicine. 318*:43

47 Cotler, M. (2000). Do Not Resuscitate Order; Clinical and Ethical Rationale and Implications, The *Medicine and Law* 19(3), 623-634.

48 Rien de Vos, Hanneke, de Haes, Koster and deHaan, (1999). Quality of survival after cardiopulmonary resuscitation. *Archives of Internal Medicine. 159* pp. 249-254.

third of the surviving patients ranging from memory deficits to a persistent vegetative state. A study was undertaken among patients admitted to the Department of Rehabilitation for Neurological Impairments at Pitié-Salpêtrière in Paris following cerebral anoxia after cardiac arrest between 1995–2007 to delineate the resultant neurological sequelae. Peskine et al. found that fourteen of the thirty patients in the study presented with severe disability and sixteen patients presented with moderate disability.[49] In the group with severe disability, no patients were autonomous for daily life activities and 64% of them presented with motor disorders. In the group with moderate disability, patients were autonomous in daily life and had no motor impairment, but could not do complex activities or functions and suffered from executive and memory impairments.[50] The potential cognitive outcomes from CPR should be addressed with the patient by the medical team during the informed consent process.

Quality of life after resuscitation may also be impacted by the aforementioned violence of resuscitation which might include skin burns, broken ribs, and stomach injuries as the side effects of defibrillation and chest compressions, even when properly performed. Although the American Heart Association correctly observes that fear of complications should not prevent one from providing CPR, these complications are part of an analysis of the burdens and benefits of CPR. This speaks directly to the patient's quality of life which should be considered along with the small probability of survival when trying to determine if the use of CPR is warranted. The non-death negative outcomes of CPR can be a significant concern within the general DNR discussion, the ethical implications of which we will now examine.

---

49 Peskine, A., Rosso, C., Picq, C., Caron, E., & Pradat-Diehl, P. (2010). Neurological sequelae after cerebral anoxia. *Brain Injury,24*(5), 755-761. doi:10.3109/02699051003709581

50 Ibid.

Classical Utilitarian Philosophy—Basic Tenets

There are many schools of thought in the broad scope of utilitarianism, but this paper will focus on classical or act utilitarianism. Act utilitarianism holds "that an act is right if its consequences are at least as good as those of any alternative," which can be directly applied to CPR and DNR.[51] Frey considers act utilitarianism to be consequentialist, aggregative, and maximizing in nature which is in line with the principle of utility as espoused by John Stuart Mill. Mill's theory of utilitarianism focuses on the utilitarian goal of maximizing pleasure and avoiding pain. According to Mill, "actions are right in proportion as they tend to promote happiness, wrong as they tend to produce the reverse of happiness."[52] Mill also considers pleasure or happiness to be an aggregate pleasure of everyone involved in a situation which, in the case of DNR or CPR, would include the patient, the patient's family and friends, the physician, other medical personnel, and, to a limited extent, the community as a whole. This thought is based on Mill's statement that "[n]o person is an isolated being" which implies that happiness is an aggregate happiness of everyone affected by the action.[53] One can readily see that the quantitative and qualitative aggregate happiness/pain balance could either justify CPR or justify the withholding of CPR based on the potential patient outcomes.

---

51 Frey, R. G. (2004). Utilitarianism and bioethics. In S. Post (Ed.), *Encyclopedia of bioethics* (3rd ed.) (Vol. 5; 2531-2534). New York, NY: Macmillan Reference, p. 2531.

52 Mill, J. S. (2001). Utilitarianism. London, GBR: ElecBook. Retrieved from http://www.ebrary.com, p. 13.

53 Ibid, p. 98.

Utilitarian View of CPR and DNR

If CPR resulted in absolute recovery of all physical and mental functioning with no adverse sequelae, then the utilitarian theory would support the intervention of CPR if there is no DNR order in place. In fact, a utilitarian would furthermore support CPR that resulted in absolute recovery even if there were a DNR order in place because the outcome would provide the most pleasure and happiness for everyone involved. However, this would violate the current ethics of DNR orders and the obligation of medical personnel to honor said orders.

On the other hand, if the patient's outcome were to result in brain damage that decreases mental or emotional capacities or physical sequelae that limits function, creates pain, or inflicts suffering, as I have shown to be true, then the aggregate weight of pain and suffering would lead utilitarians to prefer to allow the patient to die naturally from the emergent situation instead of pursuing CPR. While the pain and suffering for the patient would end immediately and the family and friends' emotional pain and grief would increase in the short-term, the overall level of pain and suffering would be decreased because the patient's family would not need to see this person endure daily, unremitting suffering. Given that the happiness balance favors a natural death in these situations, one could conclude that death is preferred from the utilitarian point of view because as Ozolins argues "utilitarianism suggests that, for many people who are living lives of permanent suffering, their lives are not worth living."[54]

Thus far, the utilitarian evaluation of CPR has been considered with the understanding that the outcome was either definitively positive or

---

54 Ozolins, J. (2015). Rationality in utilitarian thought. In Ozolins J.T. & Grainger, J. (Eds), *Foundations of healthcare ethics: Theory to practice (pp. 102-119). Cambridge, UK: Cambridge University Press.*

definitively negative. However, what should one do if the outcome is not so clear cut? After all, as discussed previously, fewer than twenty percent of patients survive CPR and eventually get discharged from the hospital. That number drops to less than five percent for frail and elderly patients. Given the high morbidity and mortality rates following CPR, particularly following extended periods of anoxia, the pleasure or pain calculation suddenly becomes less clear. In fact, a utilitarian might argue that one should not engage in CPR if the outcome is highly likely to deliver future pain and suffering through the loss of cognitive and physical functioning. From a utilitarian point of view, the decision-making process for CPR would benefit from greater insight into which factors have the greatest predictive value in determining patient outcomes. Theoretically, there would need to be a greater than fifty percent chance that the potential benefit (life with quality equal to that prior to event) of CPR would outweigh the potential cost (pain, suffering, loss of intellect). Utilitarian theory dictates that the greatest happiness must be sought, so weighing all the potentiating factors becomes central to the decision making process.

Conclusion

Outcomes from cardiopulmonary resuscitation (CPR) are unfortunately quite poor. The current healthcare system has seen an overuse of CPR mainly due to unrealistic expectations, unintended consequences of existing policies, and failure to honor patient refusal of CPR. The fact that many patients with DNR orders want CPR in specific clinical scenarios, directly conflicting with their documented DNR status is a sign that the decision-making process is unclear and the discussion about DNR is lacking in clarity and specificity.[55] According to Jesus et al., DNR orders do not accurately represent patient preferences across a variety of clinical scenarios with patients most likely to prefer to deviate from their DNR order when there is a corresponding high degree of condition reversibility.[56] Given the uncertainty of the outcomes from CPR, utilitarians would necessarily support the current state of DNR and CPR. Changing to "Never resuscitate unless there is a CPR order" for hospitalized patients would mean that there would be instances where a patient could have a positive outcome from CPR, but the process would not be initiated and the patient would die. This would be directly counter to the utilitarian goal. So, getting back to our friend Hamlet, if he were to ask a utilitarian, "to resuscitate or not to resuscitate," how would a utilitarian respond? A utilitarian would advocate for the current system of "Always resuscitate unless there is a Do-Not-Resuscitate (DNR) order" as long as there is sufficient, necessary information for making the decision that creates the most happiness for everyone involved.

References

American Medical Association. (1991). Medical futility in end of life care. JAMA. 281: 937-41.

http://www.ama-assn.org/ama/pub/physician-resources/medical-ethics/code-medical-ethics/opinion2037.page?

---

55 Jesus, J., Allen, M., Michael, G., Donnino., M., Grossman, S., Hale, C., ... Fisher, J. (2013). Preferences for resuscitation and intubation among patients with do not resuscitate/do not intubate orders. *Mayo Clinic Proceedings, 8*(7), 658-665.

56 Ibid.

American Medical Association. (1991). Guidelines for the appropriate use of do-not resuscitate orders. JAMA.265(14):1868-1871. doi:10.1001/jama.1991.03460140096034.

Cotler, M. (2000). Do Not Resuscitate Order; Clinical and Ethical Rationale and Implications, The Medicine and Law 19(3), 623-634.

Ehlenbach, W., Barnato, A., Curtis, J., Kreuter, W., Koepsell, T., Deyo, R., & Stapleton, R. (2009). Epidemiologic Study of In-Hospital Cardiopulmonary Resuscitation in the Elderly. New England Journal of Medicine 361:22-31. DOI: 10.1056/NEJMoa0810245

Frey, R. G. (2004). Utilitarianism and bioethics. In S. Post (Ed.), Encyclopedia of bioethics (3rd ed.) (Vol. 5; 2531-2534). New York, NY: Macmillan Reference.

Handley, A. (2001). Do not resuscitate. Heart, 86(1), 1–2. http://doi.org/10.1136/heart.86.1.1

Jesus, J., Allen, M., Michael, G., Donnino., M., Grossman, S., Hale, C., ... Fisher, J. (2013). Preferences for resuscitation and intubation among patients with do not resuscitate/do not intubate orders. Mayo Clinic Proceedings, 8(7), 658-665.

Mill, J. S. (2001). Utilitarianism. London, GBR: ElecBook. Retrieved from http://www.ebrary.com

Ozolins, J. (2015). Rationality in utilitarian thought. In Ozolins J.T. & Grainger, J. (Eds), Foundations of healthcare ethics: Theory to practice (pp. 102-119). Cambridge, UK: Cambridge Univ. Pr.

Peskine, A., Rosso, C., Picq, C., Caron, E., & Pradat-Diehl, P. (2010). Neurological sequelae after cerebral anoxia. Brain Injury,24(5), 755-761. doi:10.3109/02699051003709581

Rien de Vos, Hanneke, de Haes, Koster and deHaan, (1999). Quality of survival after cardiopulmonary resuscitation. Archives of Internal Medicine. 159 pp. 249-254.

Rozenbaum, E. & Shenkman, L. (1988). Predicting Outcomes of In-Hospital Cardiopulmonary Resuscitation. Critical Care Medicine.

Shakespeare, W. & Froumentin, M. (2001). The tragedy of Hamlet, Prince of Denmark. Retrieved from https://www.w3.org/People/maxf/XSLide-

Maker/hamlet.pdf

Tomlinson T. & Brody, H. (1988). Ethics and communication in do not resuscitate orders. New England Journal of Medicine. 318:43

Van Delden, J. J. M. (2012). Do-not-resuscitate decisions. In D. Callahan, P. Singer, & R.

Chadwick (Eds.), Encyclopedia of Applied Ethics (Second Edition). (pp. 859-865). doi:10.1016/B978-0-12-373932-2.00137-X

Case Study

Marvin presents to the Emergency Department with colicky flank pain and hematuria. After a noncontrast CT scan shows an eight millimeter stone in his left ureter, he is admitted to the hospital under the care of the urology service. The CT scan also showed a pancreatic head mass which, after further work-up during the hospitalization, was diagnosed as pancreatic adenocarcinoma.

You are a surgical oncologist called to consult on the case. You go to Marvin's room to discuss the diagnosis and explain that pancreatic cancer is a very deadly disease, and that Marvin's only real hope for any long-term survival is to undergo pancreatoduodenectomy (aka Whipple procedure) soon. You also explain that Marvin's chances for survival are slim even with the surgery and that the operation carries significant risk for morbidity. Nevertheless, you remind him that without the operation his chance for survival is essentially nil and you strongly recommended that he have the surgery as soon as possible while the tumor is still operable.

After listening to your recommendations, Marvin, who is 72 years old, tells you that he understands that he has no chance of survival without the surgery, and a slim chance with it. Marvin explains that he is a man of faith, and that he is ready to meet his maker that he has lived a full life, and that he has got no regrets. He goes on to say that he does not want to spend his last days in a hospital recovering from surgery just to add a year or two to his life and that he prefers to choose quality of life over quantity of life.

Marvin's wife and two grown children, who are present, begin to argue with him and urge him to reconsider. However, Marvin remains peacefully steadfast that he does not want the operation. You inform the family you will return the next day to follow up.

Ethical Questions to Ponder

(1) What do or should you suggest to the family before you leave the patient's room?

(2) What stance do you take the following day when you return to see the patient? Why?

(3) Do you have an obligation to advocate for surgical intervention because of the slim chance of increased survival?

(4) Should the plea from Marvin's family influence your advocacy for intervention if the physician personally can understand and even respect Marvin's decision?

(5) What effect will your own personal faith—or lack thereof—have on your respect for and understanding of the patient's faith-based decision making?

Chapter 5

Policy and Practice
Chicken and Egg

From an ethical perspective, with a special emphasis on vulnerable populations, this chapter explores the scope of health policy, policy options, and policy making at societal and institutional levels. This will also include examination of what ethics can and should contribute to health policy and its development.

Public health ethics or health policy ethics when viewed as determining what we ought to do in pursuit of the good of public health is an unavoidably necessary consideration in a comprehensive consideration of medical ethics. The topic is complicated by the fact that ethics appears more concerned with theoretical reflections, whereas health policies direct concrete courses of action. However, ethics loses its purpose if it does not guide specific, practical policies. Moreover, ethically sound health policy is likely to be a practical, effective health policy.

Discussion Topics

Ethics in Health Policy

Jim Summers, in "Theory of Healthcare Ethics," presents a comprehensive overview of the philosophical theories that might be applicable
to healthcare ethics.[01] Summers acknowledges that some of the theories
are not very useful in the field of healthcare ethics while others are among
the most commonly used. In toto, these theories combine to form what
Summers calls an ethics toolbox.[02] The discussion of authority-based
ethics, which can be religious, cultural tradition, or ideological in nature,
is particularly interesting because the theories are so hard to apply, but
people believe so strongly in those theories that we eventually need to deal
the ethics implications. As Summers states, "patients often have religious
views that can help them to understand and cope with their condition.
Understanding a person's faith can help the clinician provide health care
that is more patient focused."[03] Some patients see respect for their religious views as an ethical issue. Those patients may deem a clinician who
does not have requisite respect for religious views as potentially lacking
in respect a patient's right to beneficence, nonmaleficence, autonomy,
and justice. So, while authority-based ethics might not be applicable in
an overarching, normative manner to healthcare ethics, there is a role for
religion, traditions, and ideology in clinical practice.

Summers' chapter, "Principles of Healthcare Ethics," covers the four
main principles that must apply to all patients and are at the core of clin-

---

01 Summers, J. (2014). Theory of healthcare ethics. In E. Morrison, & B. Furlong (Eds.),
Health care ethics (pp. 3-45). Burlington, MA: Jones & Bartlett.

02 Ibid.

03 Ibid, p. 8.

ical practice and healthcare ethics: beneficence, nonmaleficence, autonomy, and justice.[04] Interestingly, even though beneficence and nonmaleficence are generally the two most well-known of the principles, Summers spends the majority of his time discussing justice.[05] In the entirety of the chapter, autonomy gets the least attention, but remains one of the more de rigueur concerns within healthcare ethics today. In the past, patients were more content to defer to the clinical expertise of their physician in a paternalistic manner of care, but nowadays that has morphed into a more equal patient-provider partnership. This becomes more complicated when dealing with patients who can be considered vulnerable populations whether due to being economically disadvantaged, a racial or ethnic minority, uninsured, low-income children, elderly, homeless, or severely mentally handicapped. We must take every measure to ensure that those patients are competent to go through the informed consent process free from coercion and if they are not competent, then we must ensure they have an appropriate surrogate to represent the patient's best interests. At the end of the day, autonomy is one piece of the principle mosaic that must work together for ethical healthcare.

Sick around America

Reid, in his documentary, *Sick around America*, focuses primarily on the problems presented by falling through the cracks in the healthcare system when a person has poor or non-existent insurance coverage and extraordinary healthcare circumstances arise.[06] The anecdotes in the doc-

---

04 Summers, J. (2014). Principles of healthcare ethics. In E. Morrison, & B. Furlong (Eds.), *Health care ethics* (pp. 47-62). Burlington, MA: Jones & Bartlett.

05 Ibid.

06 Reid, T.R., Correspondent. (2009). PBS: Sick around America. View film/media here: http://www.pbs.org/video/1099857730/ (Links to an external site.)Links to an external site.

umentary effectively point out how financially and physically devastating a disease or injury can be when one lacks adequate medical coverage. The documentary does not examine any social characteristics that might play a role except for any implicit meaning behind the anecdote about working for a company like Microsoft that covers all employees equally at no expense to the employees.

This is also addressed by Patel and Rushefsky when they examine the uniquely "American mix of public and private insurance programs... [that]...covers about 85 percent of the population but leaves over 40 million people without any insurance at all [and] leaves a portion of the population underinsured and vulnerable to catastrophic medical expenses."[07] However, Patel and Rushefsky focus their discussion on disadvantaged individuals based not only on insurance status, but also on the individual being poor, a minority, female, or other social factors.[08] The information they present shows a compelling case for correlation, but not necessarily for causation.

This is one of the points conceded by Almgren in his discussion of disparities in healthcare. He acknowledges that in "the conceptualization and methods used to investigate disparities in health care [m]uch of the literature on disparities in health care confuses correlation with causality."[09] Aside from that concession, Almgren weighs in very heavily that "disparities in U.S. health care system exist on the basis of a wide variety of social characteristics associated with other forms of social oppression and disadvantage."[10] The use of the word "oppression" seems to be an im-

---

07 Patel, K. & Rushefsky, M.E. (2014). *Healthcare politics and policy in America*. Armouk, NY: M.E. Sharpe. Chapter 6—Falling through the safety net: The disadvantaged (pp. 203-234).

08 Ibid.

09 Almgren, G. (2013). *Health care politics, policy, and services*. New York: Springer. Chapter 6 - Disparities in health and health care (pp. 243-283).

10 Ibid.

plication of willful intent as opposed to the result of systemic structures and processes. Later in the chapter, Almgren does explicitly define institutional racism as "institutional-level structures and processes that sustain the mechanisms of racial oppression with or without individual-level awareness or malicious intent."[11] Interestingly, one point that Almgran does not pursue in his analysis is the cultural impact on health. He notes that "a principal casualty of the socio-cultural genocide that accompanied the European conquest involved the elimination of ancient ways of food production, acquisition, and consumption that functioned together as crucial protective factors against diabetes."[12] Studies have shown that many diets, particularly Asian and Mediterranean diets, have better health impact than the average American diet, especially the African-American and Latino diets. Not accounting for the cultural impact of diet on healthcare outcomes is a significant flaw in the analysis of healthcare disparities.

Social Justice

The work of Powers and Faden puts several of my thoughts on justice, sufficiency, and systematic disadvantage into a structured, written argumentation. While the theory that Powers and Faden put forth is, as they themselves concede, more expansive and "less fixed by guideposts" than other theories, the authors make several points that we can apply to developing and refining public healthcare theory and policy. The applicability of the theory is particularly true regarding the portion about sufficiency. I strongly agree with the statement that "sufficiency of well-being, not

---

11 Ibid.

12 Ibid.

equality of well-being, is the central aspiration of justice ..."[13] I believe that the discussion about equity in healthcare sometimes gets off track because the people in the discussion fail to clearly identify the specific goal of the policy. What do we mean by universal healthcare? Do we expand the discussion, as Powers and Faden do, to include non-medical, non-healthcare determinants of well-being, such as food, housing, and respect? How do we account for situations where people are provided the means to achieve healthcare equity, but through autonomy and volition fail to do their part to achieve the ends of healthcare equity?

If we are to pursue Powers and Faden's "unified theory of well-being and its relation to the primary social determinants," then we must pay "attention to the causal pathways that influence the outcomes that matter centrally to justice."[14] One cannot possibly find a solution to a problem (healthcare equity) until one finds the root cause of inequity. One must tease out the factors that are correlational versus causational and not confuse one for the other. I think through exposure to and knowledge of public health theory and policy one can grow similar to the way the apostle Paul uses the milk and meat analogy in 1 Corinthians and Hebrews to describe spiritual growth and understanding.

Ethical Basis of Justice

Since a universal consensus on distributive justice will remain elusive because we live in a pluralistic society, the society in question must rely on a fair process by which to evaluate healthcare questions and arrive at equitable decisions. Gunnar Almgren argues that "the 'Justice as Fairness'

---

13 Powers, M., & Faden, R. (2006). Justice, Sufficiency and Systematic Disadvantage. *Social justice: The moral foundations of public health and health policy.* (pp. 50- 79). New York, NY: Oxford University Press, p. 51.

14 Ibid, p. 69.

Liberal theory of John Rawls [is] the optimal framework for the analysis of just health and health care policies."[15] However, Rawls's theory of justice as fairness was originally designed to be applied to the basic structure of society and not specifically to address health and healthcare.[16] While Almgren addresses this flaw and points out that Norman Daniels refines Rawls' theory to include health and healthcare, Almgren does not consider using Daniels' theory as the basis for the rest of the book *Health Care Politics, Policy and Services*, and services. This is a bit curious because Almgren believes that over time philosophical theories get modified, enhanced and improved by the next generations of theorists.

Another concept discussed in the reading that caught my attention is the concept that justice in healthcare means that each society must meet healthcare needs fairly under reasonable resource constraints. Even a wealthy, egalitarian country with a highly efficient healthcare system will need to establish limits to the healthcare guaranteed to members of the society. If people could agree on the principles of distributive justice that would determine how to set fair limits to the provision of healthcare, then the society could evaluate healthcare practices and decisions and change those that are deemed unjust. Unfortunately, as Powers and Faden argue, "plausibility of articulating universally applicable standards for evaluating well-being...is inevitably ethnocentric, while others may conclude that any recommendation of the use of such a list across cultures is a form of moral imperialism."[17] This is a weakness of the Rawlsian theory that must be acknowledged and taken into consideration when making public health policy determinations because you might end up tilting at

---

15 Almgren, G. (2012). Health care politics, policy and services: A social justice analysis, Second Edition. Springer Publishing Company. Kindle Edition.

16 Ibid.

17 Powers, M. & Faden, R. (2008). Social justice: The moral foundations of public health and health policy (Issues in Biomedical Ethics). Oxford University Press. Kindle Edition.

windmills if you try to attain a theoretical ideal in a flawed real world environment.

Strengths and weaknesses of, and greatest threats to, Medicare, Medicaid, and private insurance systems in the U.S.

Covering Medicare, Medicaid, the Patient Protections and Affordable Care Act, and private, commercial insurance from inception to possible future iterations creates a frustrating picture of the morass that is our healthcare system. When considering the good, the bad, and the ugly, taking a look at the strengths and shortcomings of each of these public programs as well as private insurance is instructive as we consider what the future face of healthcare provision should be in the U.S.

The Medicare program, which is federally funded, covers people age sixty-five and older as wells as persons younger than 65 who have disabilities or end-stage renal disease. For many elderly individuals, Medicare has changed the economics of retirement, allowing those close to the poverty line to stay above it. Another benefit of the program is its portability. With the exception of some Medicare managed care products, Medicare beneficiaries can expect to live wherever they wish and know that their benefits will stay with them. Also, relative to commercial insurance, it costs considerably less to provide coverage through Medicare. This is due in large part to the tremendous difference in administrative costs. Administrative costs for government programs hover around five percent, but can range from twelve to thirty percent for commercial insurance.[18]

One of the downsides of Medicare is trying to achieve cost savings by typically underpaying healthcare providers for their services. This causes

---

18 Patel, K. & Rushefsky, M.E. (2014). Medicare, Healthcare for the elderly. *Healthcare politics and policy in America*. Armouk, NY: M.E. Sharpe. Kindle Edition.

providers to look to commercial insurance to cover the gap, adding to the cost of private insurance coverage. One of the biggest drawbacks of the Medicare program relates to its financing, which is partially through payroll taxes. There is a concern that as the baby boomer generation retires the program will no longer be sustainable because those drawing benefits will outnumber those funding the program. This is a very valuable program that may become unviable in the future if finding, reimbursements, and costs are not restructured. Patel and Rushefsky note "questions about the long-term viability of the program. The trust fund...is predicted to be depleted by 2024 and to be inadequately funded through 2021."[19]

Medicaid is an entitlement program that provides health insurance to low-income and medically vulnerable people. States administer the program under broad federal guidelines specifying minimum coverage standards. Unlike Medicare, which is funded entirely at the federal level, Medicaid funding is shared by the federal and state governments. Perhaps the best aspect of Medicaid is its ability to extend a crucial healthcare safety net to those who would likely have no means to pay for healthcare coverage. Medicaid helps ensure disadvantaged children and low-income pregnant women have access to healthcare. Medicaid also allows states to tailor the benefits provided to meet the needs of the local population and respond to new health problems that might emerge.

One downside of Medicaid is the lack of portability. Because eligibility, benefits and reimbursement structures differ among states, it is not possible for a person covered by Medicaid to relocate to another state and maintain coverage. As states have broadened their Medicaid umbrellas to cover additional groups as a result of ACA, enrollment and, subsequently, healthcare costs have grown. This growing healthcare cost also makes Medicaid subject to cuts in reimbursement which results in many provid-

---

19 Ibid.

ers not accepting Medicaid patients thereby limiting patient options and forcing overutilization of emergency departments for primary care needs.

Assuring a just system of resource allocation - special challenges of policy making at government and private sector levels and some policy solutions.

Even a superficial comparison of the American healthcare system to those of the rest of world shows how different the systems are in form and function. Gunnar Almgren describes the American healthcare system as "a highly complex and often volatile mixture of free enterprise, philanthropy, and public sector health care."[20] The structural complexity of the American system creates numerous problems for managing the cost and allocation of resources both on the government level and the private sector, or market, level.

One of the main challenges faced by the government when creating healthcare policy is that regulation causes a price escalation effect. Consumers of healthcare tend to use more healthcare when the care is free or lower priced than market value. While this process avoids cost in a portion of society, there is a corresponding increase in overall cost and a decrease in the just distribution of healthcare resources.

An effective way to combat the over-utilization of healthcare resources by people who are receiving the care would be to charge a nominal fee for services. The amount of the fee should be similar to, but proportionally lower than, those deductibles and copays charged to participants in employer-based plans. This should create a significant enough barrier to prevent abuse of the system, but not prevent people from obtaining care

---

20 Almgren, G. (2013). The contemporary organization of health care: Health care services and utilization (pp. 161-206) *Health care politics, policy, and services*. New York: Springer. Kindle Edition, p. 161.

when absolutely necessary.

The private sector is challenged by the fact that it includes third party insurance companies as a vehicle for collecting and distributing financial transactions across the healthcare system. This presents a problem because insurance companies have shareholders and are by nature for-profit entities. Because the insurers need to make a profit, they create added expense to a system that would benefit from having as little overhead as possible.

Ideally, the private sector should opt for a government-managed third party system that functions as a non-profit with legislatively restricted administrative costs. Because the government has a fiduciary responsibility to promote the welfare of society, by handling the financial transactions for the healthcare system, the overall cost of the system would be decreased. With decreased cost, people would be able to afford more healthcare and, therefore, society would potentially see a more just allocation of resources.

At some point Americans need to come together to dramatically change the healthcare system. We need to take dramatic steps to right the ship and no longer be the country that "allocates more of its economic output to health care than all other countries, [but remain] significantly below the OECD average in the hospital and physician resources available to provide health care to its citizens."[21] Brave policy decisions need to be made to ensure we have just allocation of resources across society.

I absolutely believe that there are justice issues in America's current healthcare system. As a nation, we have some groups of people within our society who lack proper access to care because they live in a place that has no medical care within a reasonable distance. This is especially true

---

21 Almgren, G. (2013). The contemporary organization of health care: Health care services and utilization (pp. 161-206) *Health care politics, policy, and services*. New York: Springer. Kindle Edition, p. 161.

of people living in rural areas where healthcare facilities are few and far between because the population base is too low to support the fixed cost of building and running a hospital or even a clinic. Medical providers also often avoid rural areas in favor of practicing in urban or suburban areas for a multitude of reasons including financial, lifestyle, proximity to family, type of practice, etc.[22] Aside from the current process of loan forgiveness, Chan et al. as well as other researchers point to recruiting future physicians from rural populations as a way to alleviate the shortage. However, Chan et al. conclude in their study that, because two-thirds of new rural physicians were raised in urban areas, policy makers would best address the shortage by focusing on providing rural education to urban-raised medical students during medical training.

Other people lack access because of financial barriers. I believe that our health system actually has four groups of individuals when one considers the financial aspect of healthcare: insured who can afford to use their insurance, insured who cannot afford to use their insurance, uninsured who can afford healthcare (some might consider this group self insured), and uninsured who cannot afford healthcare. Those who cannot afford to obtain care, even if they have insurance, are the true unfortunates in our system. The poor who qualify for Medicaid are logically not unfortunate in terms of the healthcare aspect of their lives; they might even be considered fortunate compared to some. The true unfortunates are the people who pay monthly premiums for insurance they cannot afford to use. As I have seen anecdotally from my practice, for those individuals with private, non-governmental health insurance, premiums have increased, deductibles have increased, and the ability to use health insurance has decreased. This is an injustice in the system that has seemingly been

---

22 Chan, B. T. B., Degani, N., Crichton, T., Pong, R. W., Rourke, J. T., Goertzen, J., & McCready, B. (2005). Factors influencing family physicians to enter rural practice: Does rural or urban background make a difference? *Canadian Family Physician*, *51*(9), 1247.

exacerbated by ACA.

Thus, I believe financial reform is crucial to increasing the level of justice within the healthcare system. As Milton Friedman says in the title of his book, tells us, "there is no such thing as a free lunch."[23] The meaning behind this is that even if there is no overt price for something, there will inevitably be a hidden cost. For those on Medicaid or similar free to low out-of-pocket insurance, they are getting something for nothing because someone previously got nothing for something; people paid into the system, but got no healthcare in return. Ideally, a healthcare system would function in such a way that each individual would be incentivized to use the amount of care required to maintain health, but deterred from using more than is required. For instance, a person would benefit from getting early care for an upper respiratory infection, instead of crossing their fingers and hoping they become well before the situation ends up progressing to the point where hospitalization is required. On the other hand, we want to provide disincentive to people who opt to got to the ED instead of a PCP for a cold because the copay is $0 for each avenue of care, but the PCP requires an appointment or longer wait time. Both scenarios increase cost to the healthcare system and use resources that could and should have been avoided. Those resources and dollars could have been utilized elsewhere to increase the healthcare benefit for others within the system. Therefore, by addressing the financial underpinnings of the healthcare system, we can increase the justice and equity within the system.

The progress of health care reform efforts in the U.S. during the last century and how they were surmounted or not surmounted by Congress in 2010 and the Supreme Court in 2012

---

23 Friedman, M. (1975). *There's No Such Thing as a Free Lunch*, Open Court Publishing Company.

Politics and policy making may be the most difficult aspects of public health for a healthcare professional to manage. Clinical practice is far more straightforward, even with medical ethics thrown in, than the political gamesmanship that has taken place within healthcare reform over the last century in America. I am much more comfortable with the pursuit of justice and equity in healthcare through rational discussion and debate than wading through the political machine. I came away from this week's readings with a better understanding that Medicare Part D and ACA are actually typical of the ineffectual political process rather than unusual.

As Gunnar Almgren contends, "the policy alternatives that are most likely to be implemented are those that serve the overlapping interests of the most powerful stakeholders. Conversely, the policy alternatives that are least likely to be implemented are those that conflict with these overlapping interests."[24] This stakeholder influence results in healthcare policy that lacks efficacy and efficiency because of the vast amount of compromise necessary just to get the legislation to pass. Just to get ACA "through Congress required one compromise after another."[25] One cannot expect ACA to provide a significantly increased level of healthcare justice and equity given the immense compromise. Thomas Miller went so far as to call the passage of ACA "winning ugly."[26] The difficult experience of ACA does not bode well for the future of legislation. Over the next few decades, each of the future presidential elections will most likely include one side that want to repeal ACA and the other side that want to expand ACA.

---

24 Almgren, G. (2012). Historical evolvement of the U.S. health care system. *Health care politics, policy, and services*. (pp.49-107). New York: Springer.

25 Moore, J. (2010). Presidents and health reform: From Franklin D. Roosevelt to Barack Obama. *Health Affairs, 29*(6), 1099.

26 Miller, T. (2010). Health reform: Only a cease fire in a political one hundred years war. *Health Affairs, 29*(6), 1105.

While attempts to implement wide ranging healthcare policy were often frustrated over the last century, ACA was able to make some headway for the first time since Medicare and Medicaid were implemented. We can only wait to see if this will serve as a platform to expand the reach of healthcare justice and equity to those vulnerable patients in American society by fixing the flaws within ACA or if ACA will be repealed and replaced by new legislation and head in a completely different direction.

Intersections among social justice, public health, and communities

Good News in American Medicine, a 2012 PBS documentary, had a few interesting points dispersed throughout what felt like a propaganda piece. While we are seeking changes to the healthcare system that will provide social justice and equity to every member of society, the answers are not nearly as simple as T. R. Reid pretends they are.[27] As we have learned through the study of medical ethics and public health, not all communities can be treated the same way if we want to get outcomes that are just and equitable. The approach to healthcare in minority communities...the communication, the follow up, the therapies, the barriers to access, the reception by the community...all differ from community to community across the country. In healthcare terms and particularly in terms of the evaluation of ACA, the pursuit of social justice and equity must secure and maintain a level of healthcare sufficient for each individual to not be at a disadvantage compared to the rest of society.[28]

When we try to push public health initiatives forward, we must not only gain consensus on how we define societal obligations for social

---

27 Reid, T.R., Correspondent. (2012) PBS: Good news in American medicine.

28 Powers, M., & Faden, R. (2008). *Social justice: The moral foundations of public health and health policy.* New York, NY: Oxford University Press.

justice in healthcare, but also how to equitably allocate scarce healthcare resources and how to organize and fund healthcare systems.[29] We saw this occur during, and even after, the ACA bill was debated and became law. Today we are still debating whether ACA is salvageable or if it needs to be repealed and replaced by a new healthcare reform law.

The debate over ACA makes the information in the video even more specious as a "new" answer to healthcare reform. The free clinics frequented by those with no insurance have existed for over fifty years and are called Community Health Centers (CHC). The original intent of the CHCs was "to reduce or eliminate health disparities that affected racial and ethnic minority groups, the poor, and the uninsured" which is an essential aspect of achieving the public health initiative of providing healthcare equity and social justice to vulnerable populations.[30] Since their inception, the CHCs have grown in numbers to over eight thousand centers across the nation in both rural and urban settings, and serve the medical needs of twenty million Americans.[31] The ACA provided $11 billion in funding for CHCs between 2011 and 2015. This is just one example of the not-so-new information that Reid presented as cutting edge reform for healthcare in the US. There is no magic bullet or simple panacea for the healthcare woes we are experiencing in America. We need to do a lot of hard work that will differ in appearance across the country based on the community we serve.

---

29 Almgren, G. (2013). *Health care politics, policy, and services*. New York: Springer.

30 Adashi, E.Y., Geiger, H.J., & Fine, M. D. (2010). Health care reform and primary care— The growing importance of the community health center. *N Engl J Med* 362:2047-2050. DOI: 10.1056/NEJMp1003729

31 Adashi, E.Y., Geiger, H.J., & Fine, M. D. (2010). Health care reform and primary care— The growing importance of the community health center. *N Engl J Med* 362:2047-2050. DOI: 10.1056/NEJMp1003729

Essay 9

MORE THAN JUST INSURANCE: THE PATIENT PROTECTION AND AFFORDABLE CARE ACT INVESTMENT IN COMMUNITY HEALTHCARE

Introduction

Because the United States is a pluralistic democratic republic, political and social processes are subject to the vicissitudes wrought by the influence of disparate political parties, societal associations, and pressure groups that hold diverse points of view. The vicissitudes endemic in the nation's politics and policy making processes have a dramatic impact on the pursuit of social justice and equity in public health. Those trying to push public health initiatives forward must not only gain consensus on what are societal obligations for social justice in healthcare, but also how to equitably allocate scarce healthcare resources and how to organize and fund healthcare systems.[32] Despite being handcuffed by pluralism, the American government has repeatedly tried to solve the public health dilemma for more than a century now with the latest attempt being the Patient Protection and Affordable Care Act of 2010 (ACA). Most of the attention received by ACA has been for the changes brought to the healthcare insurance landscape across the nation. However, this paper will focus on ACA's provision for investment in the expansion of community health centers and the National Health Service Corps, which, while less well-known, will have a profound effect on medically underserved populations across the nation and help to increase justice

---

32 Almgren, G. (2013). *Health care politics, policy, and services*. New York: Springer.

and equity in the provision of healthcare in American society.

Social Justice and Equity for Vulnerable Populations in Healthcare

Before a discussion of ACA can proceed with any clarity, the framework within which ACA will be analyzed must be established. For this paper, the primary consideration is the impact of ACA on social justice and equity of healthcare provision to vulnerable populations. To borrow from Patel and Rushefsky, some people are disadvantaged within the healthcare system and specific, focused efforts should be made to overcome those disadvantages.[33] Disadvantaged individuals, who can also be called vulnerable populations, are determined to be such based on falling into one or more of the following categories or statuses: minority, older, poor, underinsured or uninsured, lack of access to care, no or few healthcare providers. Actively overcoming these disadvantages or making additional effort to provide equal care to vulnerable populations can be considered the pursuit of both equity and social justice.[34] Equity and social justice are "concerned with only those dimensions of well-being that are of special moral urgency because they matter centrally to everyone, whatever the particular life plans and aims each has."[35] Put in healthcare terms and particularly in the evaluation of ACA, the pursuit of social justice and equity must secure and maintain a level of healthcare sufficient for each individual to not be at a disadvantage compared to the rest of society.[36] Now,

---

33 Patel, K. & Rushefsky, M. (2014). Healthcare Politics and Policy in America: 2014. Taylor and Francis.

34 Ibid.

35 Ibid, p. 15.

36 Ibid.

the paper can move on to a discussion of the aspects of the healthcare system that are impacted by ACA and an evaluation of the implications for social justice and equity.

Community Health Centers (CHC)

The Community Health Centers Program (CHC) started after a physician named H. Jack Geiger went to South Africa and saw the tremendous positive impact that community-based healthcare had on the health of the poorest members of that society. Upon returning to America, Dr. Geiger joined other healthcare providers in the submission of proposals to the federal Office of Economic Opportunity to create health centers in the "medically underserved inner city and rural areas of the country based on the same healthcare model Geiger studied in South Africa."[37] The first CHCs grew out of those proposals and the War on Poverty initiatives of President Lyndon Johnson's administration in 1965 with federal funding for a facility in Boston, Massachusetts, and a facility in Mound Bayou, Mississippi.[38] The original intent of the CHCs was "to reduce or eliminate health disparities that affected racial and ethnic minority groups, the poor, and the uninsured" which is an essential aspect of achieving the public health initiative of providing healthcare equity and social justice to vulnerable populations.[39] Since their inception, the CHCs have grown in number to over 8000 centers across the nation in both rural and urban settings that serve the medical

---

37 National Health Service Corps. About us. Retrieved from http://www.nhsc.hrsa.gov/corpsexperience/aboutus/index.html

38 Ibid.

39 Adashi, E.Y., Geiger, H.J., & Fine, M. D. (2010). Health care reform and primary care — The growing importance of the community health center. *N Engl J Med* 362:2047-2050. DOI: 10.1056/NEJMp1003729, p. 2047.

needs of twenty million Americans.[40] While the CHCs are federally funded and receive some regional and local grants, CHCs need to round out their funding through "fees for services rendered to insured patients and 'pay-as-you-can' or 'sliding-scale' collections from the uninsured who account for 40% of patients served."[41] At the end of the day, CHCs serve to extend the public health goal of social justice and equity by first, never turning anyone away for lack of ability to pay and second, delivering the "primary medical, dental, behavioral, and social services to medically underserved populations in medically underserved areas."[42]

National Health Services Corps (NHSC)

The National Health Services Corps (NHSC) began in the United States in 1972 as a response to the dearth of physicians serving the medical needs of vulnerable populations in both rural and urban areas. The retirement of older physicians and the increased election by new physicians to pursue specialization instead of primary care in the 1950's and 1960's exacerbated the shortage of primary care physicians (PCPs) in underserved areas. The NHSC was specifically tasked with addressing the primary healthcare shortage by incentivizing physicians to practice in underserved areas through scholarships and loan repayment programs thereby "improv[ing] the delivery of health services to persons living in communities and areas of the United States where health personnel and services are inadequate."[43] The NHSC has now grown to

---

40 Ibid.

41 Ibid.

42 Ibid.

43 National Health Service Corps. About us. Retrieved from http://www.nhsc.hrsa.gov/corpsexperience/aboutus/index.html

over 9,200 primary care physicians who provide basic medical services to almost ten million vulnerable Americans in underserved areas of the country with no regard for the individual's ability to pay for care.[44] The NSHC is vital to the provision of healthcare in underserved areas of the country; without it, social justice and equity in public health would be difficult to achieve.

School-Based Health Centers (SBHC)

School-based Health Centers grew out of the local initiatives in New York City in the early 1900's to address the spread of communicable disease among school-aged children. Within one year the absentee rate had fallen by 90% and attention was brought to the impact school nurses could have on the health of a community.[45] Little by little, the provision of healthcare in schools spread across the country until the system eventually coalesced by the early 1980's into SBHC with presence in several states including California, Louisiana, Colorado, and New York.[46] SBHCs continued to grow spread throughout about 120 by 1988 and over 350 by the end of the 1990's.[47] As Keeton et al. point out, given that over 70% of students in schools serviced by SBHCs, "increased accessibility and continuity of health care on the school campus makes the SBHC an ideal setting for the diminishing and eventual elimination of these health disparities."[48] However, funding

---

44 Ibid.

45 Keeton, V., Soleimanpour, S., & Brindis, C. D. (2012). School-Based Health Centers in an Era of Health Care Reform: Building on History. *Current Problems in Pediatric and Adolescent Health Care*, 42(6), 132–158. http://doi.org/10.1016/j.cppeds.2012.03.002

46 Ibid.

47 Ibid.

48 Ibid, p. 7-8.

has been a continual problem for SBHCs and out of over 98,000 public schools , there are only 1900 SBHCs across the country, despite the general acknowledgement that the SBHCs play a crucial role in serving the needs of vulnerable, underserved populations.[49]

Nurse-Managed Health Clinics (NMHC)

The foundation for Nurse-Managed Health Clinics (NMHC) sprang up in the mid 1800's as a result of hospitals' inability to adequately address the needs of the poor due to lack of accessibility.[50] The NMHCs gained support from "universities as a service to the community" with a focus on "supplying clinical sites for nursing students of that specialty and providing treatment to underserved populations."[51] NMHCs eventually evolved into a fully realized vehicle for the provision of medical care and disease prevention to vulnerable patient populations with limited access to care, independent of the individual's ability to pay NMHCs provide a wide array of services to include "physical exams, cardiovascular checks, diabetes and osteoporosis screenings, smoking cessation programs, immunizations, and other prevention-focused services."[52] Health systems in America today are still confronted with serving the needs of vulnerable populations in underserved areas that lack accessibility to adequate healthcare. NMHCs help to fill that gap, but suffer from a lack of funding on the national level.

---

49 Ibid.

50 Ely, L. T. (2015). Nurse-managed clinics: Barriers and benefits toward financial sustainability when integrating primary care and mental health. *Nursing Economics. 33*:4 p. 193-202.

51 Ibid, p. 201.

52 American Association of Colleges of Nursing. Policy Briefing. (2014). Nurse-managed health clinics: Increasing access to primary care and educating the healthcare workforce. Retrieved from http://www.aacn.nche.edu/government-affairs/FY13NMHCs.pdf

Summary of Patient Protection and Affordable Care Act (ACA)

The vast majority of the Patient Protection and Affordable Care Act (ACA), signed into law by President Obama on March 23, 2010, is a comprehensive health reform aimed at expanding coverage, controling healthcare costs, and improving the national healthcare delivery system.[53] The main points of ACA that captured the nation's attention and debate include the individual mandate, the requirement for employers of 50 or more employees to offer coverage, expansion of Medicaid, premium subsidies for individuals and businesses, creation of health insurance exchanges, benefit design requirements (of particular interest is the pre-existing condition requirement), cost containment and quality measures, prevention and wellness initiatives, long-term care coverage, and, finally, other investments. This paper is focused on the impact of the items that fall under the last section called "other investment" which includes CHCs, the NHSCs, SBHCs, and NMHCs.[54] The Kaiser Family Foundation's Summary of the Affordable Care Act concisely summarizes the provisions of that section of ACA as: "Improve access to care by increasing funding by $11 billion for community health centers and by $1.5 billion for National Health Service Corps over five years (effective fiscal year 2011); establishing new programs to support school-based health centers (effective fiscal year 2010) and nurse-managed health clinics (effective fiscal year 2010)."[55] So, what does this mean for each of the entities mentioned in the above section of ACA and the impact on social justice and healthcare equity for vul-

---

53 Summary of the Affordable Care Act. The Henry J. Kaiser Family Foundation, April 25, 2013. Retrieved from http://kff.org/health-reform/fact-sheet/summary-of-the-affordable-care-act/

54 Ibid.

55 Ibid.

nerable populations?

ACA Impact on Community Healthcare Sites

With an estimated 60 million individuals classified as living in a medically underserved situation, defined as "a combination of elevated health risks and a shortage of primary healthcare professionals," one can readily see that steps must be taken to address the shortage of care.[56] ACA investment in CHCs and the NHSC is an integral and essential commitment by the federal government to address the needs of vulnerable populations who rely on the CHCs to meet healthcare needs. The $11 billion that ACA will pour into CHCs and $1.5 billion being poured into the NHSC will permit the expansion of facilities and medical staff serving those underserved communities, and is "expected to result in a doubling of the number of patients served, raising the total number of health center patients from 20 million in 2010 to approximately 40 million by 2015."[57] This type of increase in the reach of healthcare into underserved rural and urban communities cannot help but result in a commensurate increase in the overall social justice and equity of the entire healthcare system.

The potential to go unfunded has not stopped The National Association of Community Health Centers from planning for much needed growth in the future, "with a goal to serve 30 million people by 2015 and 51 million by 2022."[58] The expansion plan is highly dependent

---

56 Rosenbaum, S. (2011). The Patient Protection and Affordable Care Act: Implications for Public Health Policy and Practice. *Public Health Reports,126*(1), 130–135. Retrieved from http://www.ncbi.nlm.nih.gov/pmc/articles/PMC3001814/, p. 133.

57 Ibid.

58 Rieselbach, R.E., Crouse, B.J., & Frohna, J.G. (2010). Teaching primary care in community health centers: Addressing the workforce crisis for the underserved. *Ann Intern Med.* (152)118-122. doi:10.7326/0003-4819-152-2-201001190-00186, p. 118.

on finding enough primary care physicians (PCP) to actually staff the CHCs. The ACA provision of $1.5 billion to the NHSC for scholarships and loan forgiveness for physicians who serve in underserved areas will be a significant tool to build the PCP workforce in both rural and urban areas. According to Rieselbach et al., America currently has a need for 16,000 more PCPs to meet the staffing needs of CHCs in underserved areas.[59] The fact that ACA made provisions for funding both the CHCs and the NHSC may be an indication that there is a tacit acknowledgment of the value CHCs have in addressing the healthcare needs of poor and vulnerable populations that may fall through the cracks of ACA.

The ACA also made provisions for expansion and support of School Based Health Centers which will be essential to maintaining the stop-gap for the healthcare needs of mainly minority and poor school-aged children. According to the Health Resources and Services Administration report on SBHCs, ACA called for $200 million to improve and expand services at school-based health centers between 2010 and 2013.[60] This follows on a $95 million grant in July 2011 that allowed SBHCs to care for the health of another 440,000 children. With the ACA funding doubling that amount, one can only imagine how many more children will have increased access to healthcare services.

Conclusion

The ACA's provision for investment in expansion of the CHCs and the NHSC will have a profound effect on the medically underserved

---

59 Ibid.

60 Health Resources and Services Administration. U.S. Department of Health and Human Services. (2016). School-based Health Centers. Retrieved from http://www.hrsa.gov/ourstories/schoolhealthcenters/

and vulnerable patient population across the nation and will thereby help to increase justice and equity in the provision of healthcare in American society. The CHCs were founded to create a safety net for those vulnerable patients across the country with a focus on both "care of individual patients and on the health status of their overall target populations."[61] The dual roles of healthcare on the individual and population levels are parts of the fundamental goal for public health. The ACA may have many detractors because of the fundamental flaws the law has with regard to cost increases for many individuals, individual and employer mandates, and the large number of uninsured. However, the ACA did make sound investments in grassroots efforts to meet the needs of the most vulnerable members of the populations through funding the CHCs, NHSC, SBHCs, and NMHCs that will pay dividends into the future.

References

Adashi, E.Y., Geiger, H.J., & Fine, M. D. (2010). Health care reform and primary care—The growing importance of the community health center. N Engl J Med 362:2047-2050. DOI: 10.1056/NEJMp1003729

Almgren, G. (2013). Health care politics, policy, and services. New York: Springer.

American Association of Colleges of Nursing. Policy Briefing. (2014). Nurse-managed health clinics: Increasing access to primary care and educating the healthcare workforce. Retrieved from http://www.aacn.nche.edu/government-affairs/FY13NMHCs.pdf

---

61 National Health Service Corps. About us. Retrieved from http://www.nhsc.hrsa.gov/corpsexperience/aboutus/index.html

Ely, L. T. (2015). Nurse-managed clinics: Barriers and benefits toward financial sustainability when integrating primary care and mental health. Nursing Economics. 33:4 p. 193-202.

Health Resources and Services Administration. U.S. Department of Health and Human Services. (2016). School-based Health Centers. Retrieved from http://www.hrsa.gov/ourstories/schoolhealthcenters/

History of America's Health Centers. Retrieved from http://chchistory.nachc.org/about-community-health-centers/history-of-americas-health-centers/

Keeton, V., Soleimanpour, S., & Brindis, C. D. (2012). School-Based Health Centers in an Era of Health Care Reform: Building on History. Current Problems in Pediatric and Adolescent Health Care, 42(6), 132–158. http://doi.org/10.1016/j.cppeds.2012.03.002

National Health Service Corps. About us. Retrieved from http://www.nhsc.hrsa.gov/corpsexperience/aboutus/index.html

Patel, K. & Rushefsky, M. (2014). Healthcare Politics and Policy in America: 2014. Taylor and Francis. Kindle Edition.

Powers, M., & Faden, R. (2008). Social justice: The moral foundations of public health and health policy. New York, NY: Oxford University Press. Kindle Edition

Rieselbach, R.E., Crouse, B.J., & Frohna, J.G. (2010). Teaching primary care in community health centers: Addressing the workforce crisis for the underserved. Ann Intern Med. (152)118-122. doi:10.7326/0003-4819-152-2-201001190-00186

Rosenbaum, S. (2011). The Patient Protection and Affordable Care Act: Implications for Public Health Policy and Practice. Public Health Reports,126(1), 130–135. Retrieved from http://www.ncbi.nlm.nih.gov/pmc/articles/PMC3001814/

Rosenbaum, S. (2015), Will health centers go over the "funding cliff"?. Milbank Quarterly, 93: 32–35. doi: 10.1111/1468-0009.12103 Summary of the Affordable Care Act. The Henry J. Kaiser Family Foundation, April 25, 2013. Retrieved from http://kff.org/health-reform/fact-sheet/ summary-of-the-affordable-care-act/

Case Study

For this case, you are have an internal medicine practice in an affluent, urban location. While going about your normal morning routine, you notice that Chris, the vendor at your favorite coffee truck, is wheezing noticeably. You mention this to him and suggest that he come by the clinic after work.

Later that day when Chris presents to you in your office, you confirm that he has asthma. You take a peak flow meter reading and give him a free sample of a combined beta-agonist and steroid inhaler. Chris has no other health concerns, but states that he has no medical insurance, so he had not sought treatment when he started feeling short of breath.

You check with Chris each day when you stop for your morning coffee and notice that his breathing has improved significantly. Chris is sincerely grateful for your help and you feel a sense of satisfaction from helping him. You realize that you became a doctor to serve the needs of patients like Chris. Now you wonder how you can bridge the gap between your current practice population and the altruistic practice population that prompted you to be a doctor. So, you tell Chris to return to your office when his inhaler runs out.

The next month you give Chris another free sample. Then you notice that a few more disadvantaged people from the area have begun showing up at your office. It seems likely that Chris has told some of his friends about your pro bono work. Initially, you try to fit them in between appointments and sometimes during lunch. You provide free care and distribute samples when you have some available. You write prescriptions for medications you do not have as samples and hope that the patients can afford to fill them. You refer some patients to a local free clinic when you cannot provide the care or medication they require. However, the free clinic is known to be inefficient and difficult to access. You avoid in-depth discussions as to why these patients are uninsured or not on Medicaid, but you hypothesize that some of them are undocumented immigrants. While you cannot provide appropriate care for all of your drop-in patients, you feel that you are making a difference in the community.

A few months after first helping Chris, you realize that you have unscheduled patients in your office on a daily basis. Even though you have asked Chris not to tell anyone else about how you helped him, the flow of needy patients has not slowed. Now you are torn between wanting to help the needy patients while maintaining capacity to care for your primary patient base. Time constraints have started to become a significant issue and some of your paying patients are starting to notice the very different population in the waiting room. You want to continue caring for your indigent patients, especially the children among them, but it is becoming unsustainable.

Ethical Questions to Ponder

(1) How does one decide the amount of time one can devote to uncompensated care?

(2) At what point does one shift from standing in the gap by directly providing patient care to indirectly standing in the gap by lobbying for sweeping community policy changes to address a perceived need?

(3) How does an individual healthcare provider balance one's own "policy" with the healthcare policy of a larger organization or community?

Chapter 6

Law: When Right Is Wrong and Wrong Is Right

This chapter explores the dynamic tension between health law and health-care ethics. At times, one has difficulty discerning the point where ethics end and law begins or vice versa because that which is ethical might not be lawful and that which is lawful might not be ethical. Former Chief Justice of the U.S. Supreme Court Earl Warren described the relationship between law and ethics as follows: "In civilized life, Law floats in a sea of Ethics. Each is indispensable to civilization. Without Law, we should be at the mercy of the least scrupulous; without Ethics, Law could not exist."

Discussion Topics

Majority opinion vs. dissenting opinion

Typically, one would presume that the majority judicial opinion in a case would necessarily have the stronger argument because, by definition, the majority of the judges agreed with the finding and, therefore, support for the decision should be stronger. However, in the US Supreme Court case of *Michael H. Vs Gerald D. (1989)*, the dissenting opinion given by Justice Brennan was the stronger argument.

Justice Brennan first attacked the plurality's logic that tradition needs to be maintained in defining how relationships should be viewed in the case and which relationships demand protection. Brennan pointed to case precedents and posited that "[i]f we had looked to tradition with such specificity in past cases, many a decision would have reached a different result."[01] Brennan then proceeds to note that the Court did not ask if the interest in question was traditionally protected which "highlights the novelty of the interpretive method that the plurality opinion employs [in the *Michael H. vs. Gerald D. (1989)* case]."[02]

This leads to the sharply cutting critique by Brennan that the plurality ignored the fact that the world had changed and presumptive paternity based on marriage had been replaced by definitive blood tests. Brennan further underlined the archaic mentality behind the plurality opinion by noting that "illegitimacy no longer plays the burdensome and stigmatizing role it once did" which makes one think that the decision was being

---

01 Menikoff, J. (2001). *Law and bioethics: An introduction*. Washington, DC: Georgetown University Press, p. 116.

02 Ibid, p. 116-117.

rendered in 1889 instead of 1989.[03] Justice Brennan's argument goes a long way to show that the plurality's argument was tied to tradition in a way that bastardized the true intent of the protected relationship precedents in society.

Justice Scalia tried to rebut Justice Brennan's opinion by focusing on the semantics of "parenthood" versus "family relationship" or "personal relationship." Arguments that focus on semantics instead of foundational principles or the meaning behind the semantics come across as weak. Therefore, given the argument used by Justice Brennan, and the relatively weak counter by Justice Scalia, one must conclude that the dissenting opinion is stronger than the plurality opinion in *Michael H. vs. Gerald D. (1989)*.

Evaluation of duty between a therapist and the intended victim

With a tip of the hat to Samuel Taylor Coleridge's "Rime of the Ancient Mariner," duty duty everywhere and liability to spare. The Court decision in *Tarasoff v. Regents of the University of California* (Cal. 1976), was an example of people wanting to have their cake and eating it too. The Court believed that when a therapist or other clinician "determine[s], that his patient presents a serious danger of violence to another, he incurs an obligation to use reasonable care to protect the intended victim against such danger."[04] The court used analogous situations to support their decision such as a physician's fiduciary responsibility to guard public safety by a duty to inform a patient's family if a patient has a contagious infection or if a patient's illness or medication is likely to create a public safety

---

03 Ibid, p. 117.

04 Menikoff, J. (2001). Law and bioethics: An introduction. Washington, DC: Georgetown University Press, p. 177.

issue by impairing the operation of a motor vehicle.[05]

The Court then proceeded to acknowledge that therapists are "unable reliably to predict violent acts" by their patients.[06] The fact is that prediction is unreliable, but the Court believed that therapists should nevertheless be held responsible for notifying the potential victim or people who would reasonably notify the potential victim, putting the therapist or physician in an untenable position. The Court provides no protection for the therapist or physician from lawsuits initiated by the patient for disclosure of confidential information.

Therefore, we have a situation where a therapist has a duty to notify about a potential threat that is acknowledged to be highly unpredictable, but also has a duty to maintain patient confidentiality. So, the therapist or physician better beat the odds and be correct in notifying a potential victim or beat the odds in the other direction and make no mention of the threat in the hope that nothing happens. Failure to notify if an act is carried out will result in liability and failure to maintain confidentiality if no violent act occurs will result in liability.

The duty to protect the public is a strong argument for the creation of a duty between the therapist and the intended victim. However, the duty to protect patient confidentiality is a strong argument against the creation of a duty between the therapist and the intended victim. In light of the rock-and-a-hard-place situation in which a therapist finds herself, the Court should provide liability protection for the therapist against breach of confidentiality claims so that the therapist can notify a potential victim without fear of reprisal. Duty duty everywhere and liability to spare.

---

05 Ibid.
06 Ibid, p. 178.

The majority vs. the dissenting judicial opinions

In re Guess—Supreme Court of North Carolina 393 S.E. 2d 833 (N.C. 1990)

The majority opinion written by Justice Mitchell in the Guess case is a stronger argument than any dissenting argument based on clinical, legislative, and judicial precedents. Justice Mitchell argues that Dr. Guess was outside the boundaries of his medical practice when using homeopathy to treat patients. From a clinical standpoint, homeopathy is an alternative medical system that has received minimal support from the mainstream medical community. The National Institute of Health's (NIH) National Center for Complementary and Integrative Health (NCCIH) acknowledges that "there is little evidence to support homeopathy as an effective treatment for any specific condition" (NCCIH, 2016, Key Points).[07] This is not to say that homeopathy is not used by millions of Americans each year. However, the NCCIH goes so far as to plainly state: "Do not use homeopathy as a replacement for proven conventional care or to postpone seeing a health care provider about a medical problem" (2016, If You Are Thinking About Using Homeopathy).[08]

To further support the majority opinion, Justice Mitchell argues that homeopathy does not meet the Board of Medical Examiners' standard of "acceptable and prevailing" systems of medical practice in North Carolina as set forth by North Carolina Statute 90-14 (a)(6). The Board has the responsibility to police the medical profession's practice in order to protect the safety and welfare of the public. In this instance, the use of

---

07 National Center for Complementary and Integrative Health. National Institute of Health. (2016). *Homeopathy*. Retrieved from https://nccih.nih.gov/health/homeopathy

08 National Center for Complementary and Integrative Health. National Institute of Health. (2016). *Homeopathy*. Retrieved from https://nccih.nih.gov/health/homeopathy

homeopathy to treat an illness falls within the authority provided by the Statute because the treatment has no proven clinical value and may have some patient safety concerns.[09] The North Carolina legislature did later change the statute (NC Gen. Stat. 90-14 (a)(6) 1999) to place the onus on the Board to prove "by competent evidence, ... that the treatment has a safety risk greater than the prevailing treatment or that the treatment is generally not effective." While the revised Statute might leave the door open for the practice of homeopathy, the Statute does not completely support the practice.

Finally, the judicial precedent supports the opinion written by Justice Mitchell. Judicial judgments on the State and Federal levels have declared that states have the right to deny "patients access to a particular form of therapy or a particular type of practitioner."[10] The U.S. Supreme Court weighed in on alternative treatments and the power to police in the case of *United States v. Rutherford, 442 U.S. 544 (1979)*. The Supreme Court of the United States validated the right of the FDA to ban the use of a substance that has no proven efficacy. All of the clinical, legislative, and judicial evidence supports Justice Mitchell's majority opinion as the stronger argument.

Menikoff theoretical case about Wendy, 16, refusing cancer chemotherapy

The case for Wendy refusing chemotherapy to treat her cancer is fairly straightforward in terms of procedural factors and precedents. First, Wendy is a minor, so the onus is initially placed on her parents to make decisions about Wendy's medical care. Given that her parents "insist

---

09 Ibid.

10 Menikoff, Jerry. (2001). *Law and Bioethics: An Introduction*. Georgetown University Press. Kindle Edition, p. 213.

that [Wendy] be given the therapy," we have the first vote against Wendy making the choice to refuse chemotherapy.[11] Parental consent on behalf of a minor child is the legal norm with the child assenting to the treatment to the extent the child is developmentally capable.[12] However, exceptions to parental authority do exist including instances where there is child abuse, the parents are unavailable in an emergency situation, or the minor is emancipated.[13] Some States have statutes that allow minors to have access to care without parental consent for treatment of sexually transmitted diseases, drug dependency, mental health treatment, or for contraceptives.[14] [15]A final exception is the "mature minor" declaration, "under which minors can petition the court to recognize that they fully understand the treatments and consequences of their decisions and should therefore be allowed to make treatment decisions independently, either in contradiction to their parents' wishes or without consulting their parents."[16]

The case is not so straightforward when we look at some of the more subjective factors in the case. In Wendy's situation, one confounding factor is the relatively low, five percent chance for remission and the unpredictable and unknown duration of the remission. Courts may weigh those factors when deciding whether to support a minor's refusal

---

11 Ibid, p. 281.

12 Blake, V. (2012). Minors' refusal of life-saving therapies. *American Medical Association Journal of Ethics, 14*(10), 792-796. Retrieved from http://journalofethics.ama-assn.org/2012/10/pdf/hlaw1-1210.pdf

13 Ibid.

14 Ibid.

15 Menikoff, Jerry. (2001). *Law and Bioethics: An Introduction*. Georgetown University Press. Kindle Edition, p. 213. Ibid, p. 281.

16 Blake, V. (2012). Minors' refusal of life-saving therapies. *American Medical Association Journal of Ethics, 14*(10), 792-796. Retrieved from http://journalofethics.ama-assn.org/2012/10/pdf/hlaw1-1210.pdf, p. 793.

of medical treatment.[17] Another confounder is the lack of information about Wendy's level of maturity. If the Court determines that Wendy can be granted "mature minor" status, then the desires of Wendy's parents become irrelevant to the Court and Wendy can be granted the right to refuse medical treatment if she so desires.

The final verdict in Wendy's case seems to hinge on her status as a "mature minor." Therefore, if Wendy is determined to be a "mature minor," then she should be permitted to refuse treatment. However, if Wendy is not deemed to be a "mature minor," then Wendy's parents should have the final say and Wendy should not be permitted to refuse treatment.

In re Baby K

Several considerations combine and make the In re Baby K case more complicated than it would appear at first glance: The legal consideration of the Emergency Medical Treatment and Active Labor Act (EMTA-LA), the Americans with Disabilities Act, ethical consideration of futile medical care, and the fact that Baby K was stable for long periods of time outside the hospital.[18] Taking the into account the sum total of issues raised In re Baby K, one can certainly see that the court made the correct decision in terms of the letter of the law, but the wrong decision in terms of the clinical bioethics.

From an ethical standpoint, prolonging the life of anencephalic Baby K was wrong. Baby K's fate was certain from the moment she was born. The decision to continue to provide care for her resulted in the compromised integrity of the medical staff and most likely emotional suffering and turmoil for anyone involved with the case.

---

17 Ibid.

18 Menikoff, J. (2001). *Law and bioethics: An introduction.* Washington, DC: Georgetown University Press.

Typically, anencephaly and brain death are two clinical situations that virtually all knowledgeable clinicians agree are futile to treat. Sometimes, parents want to keep anencephalic infants alive as long as possible, but eventually come to the realization that the situation is hopeless and the family finally agrees to halt treatment. However, In re Baby K differed from the norm because Ms. H, the mother, wanted to give birth even though she knew the baby would be anencephalic and then demanded advanced life support due to religious beliefs in the "sanctity-of-life...and that God alone should decide how long the baby would live."[19] The statistics of anencephalic pregnancies and births bear out the uniqueness of Baby K's case. Upwards of 95% of the pregnancies involving anencephalic fetuses end in abortion and about 55% of the 5% that proceed to birth are stillborn.[20]

Sometimes we are confronted with the dilemma that modern medicine has advanced to the point that we can manage a patient's condition, but we might lack the understanding of where and how to determine the physical and moral limits of care. Medical ethics and a moral consensus are required to guide medical care in the future as technology pushes the treatment possibilities ever outward. The flawed decision in the Baby K case seems to indicate that legislation might be lagging behind in this area.

Henrietta Lacks

Skloot's book about the history of Henrietta Lacks and the HeLa cell line is the perfect exemplar of the legal and ethical issues presented in the other readings for this week. The Lacks story raises questions not only

19 Doyle D. (2010). Baby K. A landmark case in futile medical care. *WebmedCentral MEDICAL ETHICS, 1*(10):WMC00969 doi: 10.9754/journal.wmc.2010.00969, p. 2.

20 Doyle D. (2010). Baby K. A landmark case in futile medical care. *WebmedCentral MEDICAL ETHICS, 1*(10):WMC00969 doi: 10.9754/journal.wmc.2010.00969

about the ownership of samples given by a patient for clinical testing but also about the informed consent process. Medical samples have become more problematic because genetic research has advanced to the point that DNA from a tissue sample can be used for years, even decades, after the initial sample was taken, for purposes completely unrelated to the initial intent. Even though the material was taken from the patient and the patient is the de facto owner of the material, at what point, if ever, does the patient's interest in the material cease?

The government has yet to establish laws that set clear precedent about the ownership of biological property. At this point in time, courts have primarily ruled against the patient in cases of biological and genetic ownership. The interpretation of the courts is that once the DNA or tissue leaves the body, the material is no longer the property of the individual. The courts seem to be relying on the informed consent contracts that patients sign prior to any procedure. Unfortunately, those informed consent contracts have been poorly worded or vague in meaning. The informed consent process has become much better over time as a result of occurrences such as the Tuskegee Syphilis Study which took advantage of the test subjects' lack of knowledge and lack of resources. Eventually, the informed consent process will need to address the future use of the medical samples, given the changes in technology and the financial gain for researchers that can come from some samples. As Menikoff notes, "the law already recognizes that a reasonable patient would want to know whether a physician has an economic interest that might affect the physician's professional judgment."[21] Changing technology, patient privacy, and financial concerns all come into play and make genetics and ownership rights a complicated ethical and legal minefield.

---

21 Menikoff, J. (2001). *Law and bioethics: An introduction*. Washington, DC: Georgetown University Press, p. 409.

The connection between law and ethics

The topic of organ transplantation and how to define death provide a wonderful backdrop to illustrate the relationship between law and ethics in healthcare and medicine. The field of medicine has witnessed some amazing advances that force us to reexamine the way we evaluate situations and choices from an ethical point of view and, subsequently, from a legal point of view. The fact that a change in ethical perspective precipitates, or even forces, a change in the law is significant to understand. If we consider ethics to be the beliefs, mores, and principles that guide an individual's or a group's behaviors and actions, then we can consider law the attempt by a group or society to codify those ethics into rules as a means to control those behaviors and actions across all members. So, a change in the environment causes a reevaluation of ethical considerations of the new reality and a possible change to what the individual or group believes to be ethical behavior. Because the law was established based on previous ethical considerations, one will inevitably be confronted with a situation where the current law seems outdated in the new reality. The actors within the group or society must then use established legal mechanisms to challenge and hopefully change the laws to reflect the new reality. Therefore, ethics function as a navigator pointing the course through the world and law provides the structure to ensure we stay on course.

The lead-and-follow relationship between ethics and law is beautifully illustrated by the discussion of death in both In re Bowman and In re T.A.C.P. Both cases deal with the way that medical technology has advanced in the ares of life support and means the ares of assessing brain function. Historically, death was determined by the ceasing of breath and asystole. Then medicine advanced to the point that we could mechanically replace respiration and thereby maintain a person's heartbeat. This advance then raised the question of whether the person maintained on a respirator was actually still alive anymore. Then medicine advanced again to enable us to measure brain activity. And we as a society had to decide whether a person who was on a respirator and maintained brain activity but lacked consciousness was still alive. This evolved into the ethical debate about higher brain and brainstem function which is still going on today in certain cases. As science and medicine advanced, we had to have new discussions about the ethics of the situation and what actions we should take given our beliefs, mores, and principles. These discussions resulted in decisions that were contrary to existing laws and required legal challenges to the status quo. As In re Bowman and In re T.A.C.P. also show, the results of these ethical challenges to settled law vary from state to state, even though the argumentation is strikingly similar. In many instances, ethical perspectives might be more universal than the laws derived from the ethics.

Essay 10

THERAPEUTIC CLONING *vs.* REPRODUCTIVE CLONING: DO NOT THROW THE BABY OUT WITH THE BATH WATER

Introduction

Bill Joy, the co-founder of Sun Microsystems, wrote an article for Wired magazine in which he posited that "our most powerful 21st-century technologies–robotics, genetic engineering, and nanotech–are threatening to make humans an endangered species."[22] The mention of genetic engineering, which Joy clarified to include cloning, as a potential threat to humankind, by the former Chief Technology Officer of a computer company illustrates the level of concern cloning engenders among those at the forefront of scientific discovery. The fear of cloning's potential threats to humans is accompanied by the hope that cloning can offer humans major, significant therapeutic benefits. One can see strong similarities between the double-edge sword that is cloning and the way society has had to deal with Alfred Nobel's invention of dynamite. This paper will show that the benefits derived by society from the therapeutic applications of human cloning justify any and all ethical, legal, and social hurdles that must be confronted and overcome to prevent unethical reproductive applications of the process.

Therapeutic Cloning v Reproductive Cloning

Human cloning is the process of taking DNA material from a cell and using it to replace the DNA material in an embryo. The embryo can then journey down one of two paths. The first path is implantation into a female womb for development into a human genetically identical to the donor of the original DNA material. The second path is growth of the embryo in vitro to form stem cells which can then be differentiated into human tissue or a complete human organ. The first pathway is called reproductive cloning. This process is the creation of an exact genetic duplicate of a person from another person who already exists. Since this process was completed in 1996 with the birth of genetically identical mice, several other animals have been created using this method including

---

22 Jay, B. (2000). Why the Future Doesn't Need Us. *Wired*, 8(4). Retrieved from http://www.wired.com/2000/04/joy-2/

Dolly the sheep in Scotland in 1996, but at this time no humans have been cloned.

The second pathway of this embryonic bifurcation is called therapeutic cloning. Therapeutic cloning correlates more closely with the bioethical principles of beneficence, non-maleficence, justice, and autonomy than reproductive cloning does. From a beneficence standpoint, humans can derive fantastic benefits with few potential negative medical outcomes. The tissues derived from therapeutic cloning can be used for replacing just a few cells, such as replacing pancreatic cells in diabetes to produce insulin or replacing nerve cells in the substantia nigra portion of the brain of Parkinson's patients to produce dopamine, or even replacing entire organs such as the whole liver of a patient with cirrhosis.

Therapeutic Cloning and Principles of Bioethics

Aside from those few examples of beneficence, therapeutic cloning also provides strong arguments for being non-maleficent, increasing patient justice, and reinforcing patient autonomy. First, an organ or tissue derived from an in vitro process would obviate the need for a person, living or dead to provide an organ. This type of transplant would theoretically have no danger of rejection because the DNA would be an exact match. Also, the supply would be more reliably sourced through on-demand generation, so the recipient would not have to be placed on a waiting list for an organ. There would be no need to wait for someone to die to provide the organ that may be in less than ideal condition due to age or unknown lifestyle behaviors of the donor. Lastly, if therapeutic cloning can grow new organs as needed, then fewer people would live a life full of uncertainty and anxiety only to die waiting for an organ that never arrives.

All of these benefits of therapeutic cloning would increase justice by increasing the number of patients who can obtain a tissue or organ transplant. Healthcare equity would increase because the barriers to transplantation would be no different from the barriers for any other procedure. In fact, more people would be able to have the procedures because DNA matching would obviate the need for immunosuppressant therapy to prevent transplant rejection.

Non-maleficence would increase in case of standard organ transplantation because the pain and suffering experienced by a live donor of an organ or bone marrow would be avoided. If one considers that the embryonic cell that generated the organ or tissue would never have developed into a viable human being, then one can remove the theoretical "death" of an embryo from the non-maleficence equation. With no harm being done to any other being, the argument that therapeutic cloning is a non-maleficent process is strongly supported.

Finally, therapeutic cloning actually improves patient autonomy because patients will not have any misgivings about the procedure. The patient will not have to second guess a decision to ask a relative to donate an organ or to weigh the possibility of transplant rejection. The informed consent procedure would be much more straightforward with fewer ethical concerns for the patient to consider.

Arguments Against Cloning

Unfortunately, both therapeutic and reproductive cloning use the term "cloning" even though each procedure has very different outcomes, which can cause confusion among people debating the legality and ethics of cloning. As Lori Andrews argues, "[t]he potential physical and psychological risks of cloning an entire individual are sufficiently compelling to justify banning the procedure."[23] Furthermore, Andrews contends that "certain uses of cloning—such as creation of a clone as a source of spare organs—would likely be banned by the Thirteenth Amendment prohibition of slavery and involuntary servitude."[24] Ethical and legal considerations such as those pointed out by Andrews highlight the debate over human cloning.

In fact, both President Clinton and President Bush addressed cloning and stem cell research during their respective terms in office. After the successful cloning of Dolly the sheep in 1996 , President Clinton tasked the National Bioethics Advisory Commission to analyze the cloning process and provide guidance for potential legislation.[25] While no legislation came to fruition, the groundwork was laid for society to discuss and debate the issue of cloning. President Bush continued to press the cloning issue during his January 2003 State of the Union address in which he argued for the United States to universally ban cloning "because no human life should be started or ended as an object of an experiment, I ask you to set a high standard for humanity and pass a law against all human cloning."[26] The debate over cloning and stem cell research extends to paternity issues, but this paper will maintain the previously stated stance that the risks of cloning an entire individual are so significant that the procedure should be banned without question.

Another interesting aspect of the human cloning debate was raised by Bill Jay in his article "Why the Future Doesn't Need Us" with his theory

---

23 Menikoff, J. (2001). *Law and Bioethics*. Georgetown University Press. Kindle Edition, p. 121.

24 Ibid.

25 Ibid.

26 Roetz, H. (2006). *Cross-cultural Issues in Bioethics: The Example of Human Cloning*. Amsterdam: Brill Academic Publishers. Retrieved from http://eds.a.ebscohost.com.cuhsl. creighton.edu/ehost/ebookviewer/ebook/bmxlYmtfXzE2MDE5N19fQU41?sid=548c6d88-588b-47e2-851e-04733ebac455@sessionmgr4005&vid=0&format=EB&lpid=lp_363&rid=0

that if "we were to reengineer ourselves into several separate and unequal species using the power of genetic engineering, then we would threaten the notion of equality that is the very cornerstone of our democracy."[27] Normally, the discussion revolves around producing another exact replica of a person, but Jay twists the narrative slightly by acknowledging that scientists could theoretically manipulate a few parts of the DNA sequence and thereby change the ontology of the resultant being. While the idea that humans could evolve into separate species because of self-manipulative DNA cloning and engineering would create an interesting exercise in theoretical ethics and law, that is far afield from society's current concerns about cloning.

Conclusion

Human cloning is a scary prospect for many people. Just like Nobel's dynamite, technology can be employed to benefit humanity or destroy humanity. Are we as a species supposed to avoid biotech advances just because there is the potential for the technology to be hijacked and abused by unethical people? Just like making any medical decisions, we must balance the benefit and risk to the patient. In the case of cloning, the benefit to society far outweighs the risk, so the technology should be pursued. We must simply discuss and debate the issue on a societal level and then enact legislation to ensure that the technology can be used effectively without fear of misuse or abuse. We must be bold and courageous when pushing the boundaries of technology and venturing into new frontiers. We should not allow fear to force us to throw the baby out with the bath water.

---

27 Jay, B. (2000). Why the Future Doesn't Need Us. *Wired*, 8(4). Retrieved from http://www.wired.com/2000/04/joy-2/

References

Jay, B. (2000). Why the Future Doesn't Need Us. Wired, 8(4). Retrieved from http://www.wired.com/2000/04/joy-2/

Menikoff, J. (2001). Law and Bioethics. Georgetown University Press. Kindle Edition.

National Bioethics Advisory Committee (1997). https://bioethicsarchive. georgetown.edu/nbac/pubs/cloning1/cloning.pdf

Roetz, H. (2006). Cross-cultural Issues in Bioethics: The Example of Human Cloning. Amsterdam: Brill Academic Publishers. Retrieved from http://eds.a. ebscohost.com.cuhsl.creighton.edu/ehost/ebookviewer/ebook/ bmxlYmt-fXzE2MDE5N19fQU41?sid=548c6d88-588b-47e2-851e-04733ebac455@ sessionmgr4005&vid=0&format=EB&lpid=lp_363&rid=0

Vogel, G. (2004). Scientists take step toward therapeutic cloning. Science, 303(5660), 937-939. Retrieved from http://www.jstor.org.cuhsl. creighton.edu/stable/3836101

Essay 11

THE CASE OF ELIZABETH BOUVIA: A DIFFERENT VIEW OF SELF-DETERMINATION AND SUICIDE

Introduction

The story of Elizabeth Bouvia is one of a woman with a "complicated medical history and physical impairments [that] brings forth empathy

and concern related to the magnitude of her burden of suffering."[28] Bouvia is by all accounts a mentally competent woman, but one suffering
with quadriplegia, severe congenital cerebral palsy and degenerative, de-
bilitating, agonizing arthritis. Bouvia's health status caused her to be bed-
ridden with no opportunity for employment, so she was dependent on
the government for support and care.[29] Bouvia was eventually admitted
to Riverside Hospital where her situation became so dire and desperate
that she resolved to cease eating and starve herself to death.[30] Bouvia "re-
quested that hospital staff provide her with pain medication and hygienic
care until she died. Shortly thereafter, Riverside informed Bouvia that
when her body weight fell below a certain level, steps would be taken to
force-feed her."[31] In an effort to prevent force-feeding or discharge from
the hospital, Bouvia filed a suit against the hospital in California. In
the case *Elizabeth Bouvia v. Riverside Hospital*, the court ruled in favor
of Bouvia's position regarding hospital discharge, but ruled in favor of
the hospital regarding force-feeding. Hence, as soon as Bouvia's weight
dropped below the required level, the hospital staff started to force-feed
Bouvia. In response, Bouvia filed a first appeal which failed and then filed
a second appeal in the case *Bouvia v. Superior Court in California in 1986*
which reversed the lower court ruling. In *Bouvia v. Superior Court*, the
California Court of Appeals determined that Bouvia has the "right to re-

---

28 O'Dell, R. M. (2011). The Bouvia case revisited: An introduction to the bioethical topics
of individual rights, acts of Conscience, and the right to die. *Online Journal of Health Ethics*,
7(2). http://dx.doi.org/10.18785/ojhe.0702.05, p. 3.

29 Liang, B. & Lin, L. (2005). *Bouvia v. Superior Court*: Quality of life matters. *AMA
Journal of Ethics*, 7(2). Retrieved from http://journalofethics.ama-assn.org/2005/02/pdf/hlaw1-
0502.pdf

30 Stradley, B. (1985). *Elizabeth Bouvia v. Riverside Hospital*: Suicide, euthanasia, murder:
The line blurs. *Golden Gate University Law Review, 15*(2) pp. 407-435. Retrieved from http://
digitalcommons.law.ggu.edu/cgi/viewcontent.cgi?article=1371&context=ggulrev

31 Ibid, p. 407.

fuse medical treatment, even of the life-sustaining variety, [which] entitles her to the immediate removal of the nasogastric tube that has been involuntarily inserted into her body."[32] A person's right to refuse medical care has been an ongoing debate because of nuances that surround the issue. Variables such as the type of treatment, the mental status of the patient, the patient's prognosis, and a person's right to self-determination cloud the issue. This paper will discuss the circumstances surrounding Bouvia's case history and will argue that, contrary to the final Bouvia decision, a non-terminally ill individual, regardless of mental competence, should not be able to commit assisted suicide by refusing certain medical treatments that would prevent death.

Legal Argument Against Refusal of Care

The primary argument against a patient being permitted to refuse life-sustaining medical treatment is the State's interest in preventing suicide among the State's citizenry. Menikoff has noted that "[c]ourts and commentators have commonly identified four state interests that may limit a person's right to refuse medical treatment: [included among them are] preserving life [and] preventing suicide."[33] There have been cases such as *In re Quinlan* where a patient was terminally ill and permitted to halt medical treatments thereby allowing nature to take its course. The Bouvia case is different from cases like Quinlan because Bouvia did not have a terminal illness. Therefore, because Bouvia would survive with proper nourishment, whether self-administered or tube fed, if Bouvia were to have the feeding tube removed and eventually starved to death,

---

32 Menikoff, J. (2001). *Law and bioethics: An introduction*. Georgetown University Press, P.262

33 Menikoff, J. (2001). *Law and bioethics: An introduction*. Georgetown University Press, p. 263.

then her death would be the result of suicidal starvation. The State's right to protect the health of its citizenry from suicide has been settled law in the case *In re Caulk, 480 A. 2d 93 (1984)* which determined that a non-terminally ill person's attempt to starve to death is equivalent to attempted suicide.[34] That case also set the legal precedent that the State has the right to force-feed that person to prevent suicide.[35] Therefore, given the fact that Bouvia was not terminally ill and the State has the duty to prevent suicide, the initial court ruling to allow the hospital staff to force-feed Bouvia to prevent suicide was appropriate within the context of the situation.

Ethical Argument Against Refusal of Care

Additionally, from an ethical perspective, there is no difference between death by refusal of care and death by intentional overdose. The idea that positive and negative actions with the same result are equal has been demonstrated by James Rachels' illustrative story of Smith and Jones. Rachels tells the story of two people: in one situation, "Smith drowns his young cousin in the bathtub; in the other, Jones plans to drown his young cousin, but finds the boy already unconscious under water and refrains from saving him."[36] The intent and the outcome of the two situations presented by Rachels are the same, but Smith kills his cousin and Jones allows his cousin to die. Rachels' example leads one to logically conclude that there is no difference in certain situations between killing and allowing to die. Therefore, by extension of logic, there is no significant

---

34 Ibid, p. 264.

35 Ibid.

36 Woollard, F. & Howard-Snyder, F. (2016). Doing vs. allowing harm. In E. Zalta (Ed.). *The Stanford Encyclopedia of Philosophy*. Retrieved from http://plato.stanford.edu/archives/sum2016/entries/doing-allowing/

difference between committing suicide by taking poison or pulling the trigger of a gun and suicide by starvation through refusal of tube feeding. This again shows that the court made the ethically correct decision by not forcing the hospital staff to help Bouvia commit suicide.

Counter Legal Argument

However, one might argue that as a competent individual, Bouvia's right of self-determination supersedes the State's interests. This argument might have more credibility if Bouvia's situation were more similar to that of Karen Ann Quinlan, and if Bouvia were terminally ill. The Patient Self Determination Act of 1990 states that "an individual's rights under State law (whether statutory or as recognized by the courts of the State) to make decisions concerning such medical care, including the right to accept or refuse medical or surgical treatment" does not in actuality or intent confer the right to force a medical facility to aid and abet an individual's attempted suicide *(Section 1866(a)(1)(Q)(i) of the Social Security Act (42 U.S.C. 1395cc(a)(1))*. Therefore, one must conclude that Bouvia's right of self-determination does not extend to her specific situation.

Counter Ethical Argument

Others might agree that Bouvia would not normally have a right to engage in suicide with the assistance of the hospital staff. Those same people might say that Bouvia's situation warrants an exception because while forced tube-feeding would extend her life, that life would be unbearable and the increase in length would be negated by poor quality. This is a specious argument because one would still need to endorse not only suicide, but State-sponsored suicide assisted by the medical staff of a hospital. This would set a dangerous precedent because the hospital staff would not only need to deal with the emotional turmoil of assisting to kill someone, but also facing other patients who need to trust the staff will be able to transition from killing one patient to healing another. The ethical gymnastics required to implement Bouvia's desire for assisted suicide would severely and negatively impact the reputation of the hospital and the individual medical practitioners.

Conclusion

One can readily see that the final ruling by the appellate court in Bouvia v. Superior Court in favor of Bouvia was misguided and did not fully comprehend the underlying significance of the ruling. An individual who is not terminally ill should not be able to force a medical facility and the medical staff to play a role in her suicide. In essence, Bouvia entered the hospital under the guise of wanting medical treatment to help her situation, but ended up voluntarily creating a worse medical situation that would have caused her death and then trying to compel the doctors and nurses to not prevent her death, but rather to assist in her death. One can argue that an individual has the right of self-determination, but one cannot simultaneously argue that one has the right to force another person to violate their personal moral belief, and duties, to assist the pursuit of that right of self-determination.

References

Liang, B. & Lin, L. (2005). Bouvia v. Superior Court: Quality of life matters. AMA Journal of Ethics, 7(2). Retrieved from http://journalofethics.ama-assn. org/2005/02/pdf/hlaw1-0502.pdf

Menikoff, J. (2001). Law and bioethics: An introduction. Georgetown University Press.

O'Dell, R. M. (2011). The Bouvia case revisited: An introduction to the bioethical topics of individual rights, acts of Conscience, and the right to die. Online Journal of Health Ethics, 7(2). http://dx.doi.org/10.18785/ojhe.0702.05

Patient Self Determination Act of 1990. Omnibus Budget Reconciliation Act of 1990. ((42 U.S.C. 1395cc(a)(1)) (1990).

Stradley, B. (1985). Elizabeth Bouvia v. Riverside Hospital: Suicide, euthanasia, murder: The line blurs. Golden Gate University Law Review, 15(2) pp. 407-435. Retrieved from http://digitalcommons.law.ggu.edu/cgi/viewcontent.cgi?article=1371&context=ggulrev

Woollard, F. & Howard-Snyder, F. (2016). Doing vs. allowing harm. In E. Zalta (Ed.). The Stanford Encyclopedia of Philosophy. Retrieved from http://plato.stanford.edu/archives/sum2016/entries/doing-allowing/

Essay 12

THE CASE OF THE HAVASUPAI TRIBE: IMPLICATIONS OF IMPROPER INFORMED CONSENT

Introduction

Patients must trust that the medical provider has the best interests of the patient at heart. The patient must also trust that on both the individual and organizational levels, information that is clear, complete, and easily understood, will be provided during the informed consent process. The informed consent process becomes especially pertinent during medical research studies or during diagnostic testing of patient specimens that may also be of use in research. One case that exemplifies the latter scenario is the Havasupai Indian Tribe case which involves the gathering of blood samples by researchers at Arizona State University to search for a link to diabetes. Unfortunately, the medical team decided to use the Havasupai samples for other research including schizophrenia, migration patterns and inbreeding which violated the basic rule of human based research ethics. This issue is central to the understanding of procedures for ethical community-based participatory research and the underlying principles of informed consent. This paper discusses the ways that the Havasupai Indian Tribe case highlights the need to develop the ethical and legal framework, particularly the informed consent process, in which genetic research is conducted so as to ensure the promotion of scientific progress while protecting participants.

Background

The Havasupai Tribe entered into a research study with Arizona State University in 1989 in an attempt to find the reason behind the exceedingly high rate of Diabetes Mellitus II (DMII) among the community. One of the investigative and treatment steps of the projects was genetic testing of blood samples to look for a genetic cause for DMII, but that proved fruitless. Unfortunately, the researchers then decided to use the blood samples "for other unrelated studies such as studies on schizophrenia, migration, and inbreeding, all of which are taboo topics for the Havasupai."[37] Serendipitously, a member of the Havasupai Tribe who was also part of the DMII study learned about the use of the samples

---

37 Garrison, N. (2012). Cases of how tribes are relating to genetic research. *American Indian and Alaska Native Genetics Research Resource Guide: Tools for tribal leaders and citizens.* Retrieved from http://genetics.ncai.org/files/NCAI%20genetics%20research%20resource%20guide%20FINAL%20PDF.pdf, p. 60-61.

outside the intended study when attending a lecture at Arizona State in 2003.

The Havasupai Tribe subsequently filed a lawsuit to redress their grievances *(Havasupai Tribe of the Havasupai Reservation v. Arizona Board of Regents and Therese Ann Markow, 2004)*. The lawsuit had a lengthy list of complaints including a lack of informed consent. The case never reached a definitive end in court because the two sides reached "a settlement in April 2010 in which tribal members received $700,000 for compensation, funds for a clinic and school, and return of DNA samples."[38] While the settlement is a minor victory for the Havasupai Tribe, the fact that the settlement was reached outside the court system means that the case does not contribute a legal precedent to guide future issues regarding informed consent in medical research, especially when performed among minority and vulnerable populations.

Informed Consent

The informed consent process is central to ethical medical research and needs to be followed in order to maintain the integrity of the field and future participation. The settlement reached in the Havasupai case as noted previously, did not do much to advance the legal standing of informed consent, but only actually served to underscore the basic tenets of the Common Rule. The Common Rule requires "that the researchers describe the nature and purposes of the research, as well as both reasonably foreseeable and unforeseeable risks of participation."[39]

---

38 Ibid.

39 Vorhaus, D. (2010, April 21). The Havasupai Indians and the challenge of informed consent for genomic research. *Genomics Law Report*. Retrieved from http://www.genomicslawreport.com/index.php/2010/04/21/the-havasupai-indians-and-the-challenge-of-informed-consent-for-genomic-research/, p. 1.

The use of the word "reasonably" leaves an opening for informed consent to not be completely and fully informed. Patients will not be able to determine whether participating in the research "serves his or her best interests, aims, and values" if the decision to participate is not fully informed.[40] This is not to say that the entire weight of informed consent is on the medical provider or researcher. Aside from the provider, institutional review boards (IRB), research ethics committees (REC), state and federal legislatures, and the various courts of law play a role in fashioning an informed consent process that gives patients the chance to make decisions voluntarily and with the greatest level of knowledge possible. As Brock argues, by instituting formal requirements for full disclosure to patients, there might be an opportunity "for the investigator to share further information honestly, answering questions and identifying unanswerable questions, appreciating doubts and respecting fears."[41] This would be a positive environment for informed consent between the medical provider and the patient.

Cultural Implications

The informed consent process becomes more complicated when dealing with certain ethnic or vulnerable populations. The Havasupai Tribe had an origin story just as most populations across the globe have. The use of genetic information to analyze migration patterns and thereby speculate about the accuracy of the tribe's origin may create significant conflict with and among the members of the tribe. If the tribe's identity is tied to how their ancestors came to exist, and that story is proven false,

---

40 Brock, D. (2008). Philosophical justifications of informed consent in research. In E. Emanuel, R. Crouch, C. Grady, R. Lie, F. Miller, & D. Wendler (Eds.), *The Oxford Textbook of Clinical Research Ethics* (pp. 606-612). Oxford University Press. Kindle Edition, p. 611.

41 Ibid, p. 631.

then the entire basis for the tribe's cultural beliefs comes into question.

Another aspect brought to light by the Havasupai case is the use of genetic information to determine the level of inbreeding within a population. According to Garrison, Markow's research used an "inbreeding coefficient" to analyze the genetic pool and found that the Havasupai Tribe has a higher level of inbreeding when compared to other tribes.[42] Garrison went to explain that the inbreeding information may not have been communicated clearly to the tribe because the information was interpreted to mean that tribal members inbred within a family instead of across the tribe.[43] Familial inbreeding "for the Havasupai and for many other tribes is a taboo and people who break that taboo might have problems later in life."[44] Breaking taboos could lead to excommunication from the tribe and complete loss of identity for the individual.

Betraying the trust implicit in the informed consent process can also lead to distrust of the medical community , which carries over to future interactions. There are some tribes that still refuse to work with Arizona State University because of the Havasupai case.[45] The Tuskegee syphilis research study also had a negative long-term impact on future healthcare initiatives in that minority community. The Tuskegee study was more

---

42 Garrison, N. (2012). Cases of how tribes are relating to genetic research. *American Indian and Alaska Native Genetics Research Resource Guide: Tools for tribal leaders and citizens.* Retrieved from http://genetics.ncai.org/files/NCAI%20genetics%20research%20resource%20 guide%20FINAL%20PDF.pdf

43 Ibid.

44 Garrison, N. (2012). Cases of how tribes are relating to genetic research. *American Indian and Alaska Native Genetics Research Resource Guide: Tools for tribal leaders and citizens.* Retrieved from http://genetics.ncai.org/files/NCAI%20genetics%20research%20resource%20 guide%20FINAL%20PDF.pdf, p. 63.

45 Sterling, R. (2011). Genetic research among the Havasupai—A cautionary tale. *AMA Journal of Ethics, 13*(2) pp. 113-117. Retrieved from http://journalofethics.ama-assn. org/2011/02/hlaw1-1102.html

egregious than the Havasupai case because the researchers failed to not only inform the participants of the consequences of their illness, but they also failed to treat the participants once a cure was developed. This created community backlash and distrust of the medical establishment by the African-American community which resulted in delayed diagnosis and treatment of HIV/AIDS within that community after the disease was first identified. Trust is difficult to build and can be destroyed by one simple act of betrayal.

Barriers to Informed Consent

This is not say that informed consent and consideration of ethnic cultural mores is easy or simple to implement. This is especially true when one factors in the unknown future of genetic testing and the applications of that testing. As Garrison notes, "advances in genetic research happen all the time, so it can be hard for a researcher to predict all the possible types of research that can be done with a sample, so comprehensive inclusion in the Informed Consent documentation may be difficult to achieve."[46] This is further complicated because informed consent must be distilled into language that the patient or participant can fully understand. Barriers to understanding may limit the range and scope of a research study which may exclude some of the people who would be most vital to the success of the study. These problems can be overcome by falling back on complete and sincere adherence to the bioethical principles of beneficence, nonmaleficence, autonomy and justice.

---

46 Garrison, N. (2012). Cases of how tribes are relating to genetic research. *American Indian and Alaska Native Genetics Research Resource Guide: Tools for tribal leaders and citizens.* Retrieved from http://genetics.ncai.org/files/NCAI%20genetics%20research%20resource%20 guide%20FINAL%20PDF.pdf, p. 61.

Conclusion

The case of *Havasupai Tribe against ASU* is an exemplar of how vital informed consent is to the patient-medical provider relationship. Without proper, ethical informed consent, the patient or participant may end up feeling betrayed. This places the onus squarely on medical providers since patients are exceedingly vulnerable during medical encounters and because, even in this age of online access to medical information, the healthcare provider owns the balance of power in the relationship. The lessons learned from experiences such as the Havasupai Tribe diabetes project and the Tuskegee syphilis study underscore the importance of a rigorous informed consent process. Hopefully, legal and medical systems will be able to work together to craft a patient-centric informed consent environment.

References

Brock, D. (2008). Philosophical justifications of informed consent in research. In E. Emanuel, R. Crouch, C. Grady, R. Lie, F. Miller, & D. Wendler (Eds.), The Oxford Textbook of Clinical Research Ethics (pp. 606-612). Oxford University Press. Kindle Edition.

Garrison, N. (2012). Cases of how tribes are relating to genetic research. American Indian and Alaska Native Genetics Research Resource Guide: Tools for tribal leaders and citizens. Retrieved from http://genetics.ncai. org/files/NCAI%20genetics%20research%20resource%20guide%20 FINAL%20PDF.pdf

Havasupai Tribe of the Havasupai Reservation v. Arizona Board of Regents and Therese Ann Markow. 2004. Coconino County, Superior Court of Arizona.

Sterling, R. (2011). Genetic research among the Havasupai—A cautionary tale.

AMA Journal of Ethics, 13(2) pp. 113-117. Retrieved from http://journalofethics.ama-assn.org/2011/02/hlaw1-1102.html

Vorhaus, D. (2010, April 21). The Havasupai Indians and the challenge of informed consent for genomic research. Genomics Law Report. Retrieved from http://www.genomicslawreport.com/index.php/2010/04/21/the-havasupai-indians-and-the-challenge-of-informed-consent-for-genomic-research/

Case Study

For this case, you are a physician located in Oregon with a colleague/ friend named Dr. Sharp who is diagnosed with a terminal illness; She must close her practice and relocate across the country for treatment and family support. You offer to take on several of her patients to ease the stress of the transition.

One of the patients you accept is Michelle, a 37-year-old female with bone cancer to whom Dr. Sharp provided a great deal of emotional support in addition to medical treatment. Dr. Sharp was extremely concerned about the ongoing care provided to Michelle and phones you to follow up. During your conversation, Dr. Sharp somberly tells you that there was one task she promised she would see through with Michelle, but could not complete before her retirement. Dr. Sharp asks you to complete that task so she can have peace of mind in her retirement and focus on her treatment.

She asks you to write Michelle a prescription for secobarbitol so that she can address end-of-life and make a decision about her own death, on her own terms. After checking Michelle's chart, you notice that three physicians have certified in writing that Michelle is within six months of death and that she has been found to be mentally competent by a psychiatrist who you know and trust. You also find in her file a long, compelling letter written by Michelle detailing why she wants access to medication to end her life, how she has researched her options over the last few years, and how she willingly asked Dr. Sharp for a prescription.

You are aware that the Attorney General has encouraged the DEA to take action against physicians who participate in physician-assisted suicide. You take a great deal of time and effort to evaluate the situation with Michelle. In Oregon, under State law, Michelle meets the criteria for assistance, and you know that you will be required to record your participation and the lethal prescription of the lethal dosage of medication with the Oregon Department of Health. From a Federal law perspective, you know that the DEA has guidance to take action against you if you help Michelle. Your friends and colleagues counsel you that your duty is to the patient and the people of Oregon who approved the law by a majority vote. They also contend that Michelle has the right to make this decision and if no one helps her, then it would be the equivalent of abandoning a patient at their hour of need.

You agree that terminally ill adults have a right to death with dignity, however, you worry that the Federal government will revoke your DEA license which would impact your ability to care for other patients.

Ethical Questions to Ponder

(1) What do you do for Michelle?

(2) Is physician-assisted suicide fundamentally incompatible with a physician's role of healer?

(3) Given that Michelle will need opiate medication for adequate pain control, what are your concerns, given that about even if you do not prescribe the lethal medication, she could use the opiates to end her life?

(4) What are your thoughts DEA agents easily being able to determine the differences between intentionally causing a death and prescribing enough medication to provide adequate pain relief?

(5) How will the Attorney General's guidance to the DEA impact your decision-making as a medical professional with an important clinical and ethical role in society?

Chapter 7

Practical Ethics: Shades of Gray

Most of the common activities in clinical ethics, such as ethics consultation, policy review and development, and ethics education fall under the work of institutional or system ethics committees. One foundational aspect of the application of ethics to healthcare is the assessment of the ethical issues in a clinical case to differentiate ethics from other types of problems one encounters in a clinical setting.

Discussion Topics

Views of Non-healthcare representatives on healthcare ethics committees

I spend so much of my time physically and mentally in health care that I need to ensure my environment does not cause an echo chamber effect and prevent me from considering alternative ideas.

I eventually found two people who gave me their opinions about the purpose and function of a health care ethics committee. One was a single, Asian male with no children who is a college graduate in his late forties and works as an architect for a commercial builder. The other was a married, Caucasian mother of two girls who is a high school graduate in her late forties who works as an assistant manager for a retail mass merchandiser. I list the demographic descriptors for each person to provide personal context for the answers they gave.

I spoke to each person separately and started the discussions by asking each to define 'ethics'. Both the architect (A) and the manager (M) gave a general definition of 'ethics' as morals of right and wrong that direct decisions and actions. Both A and M have to deal with business ethics in their respective careers, but have not had any prior dealings with health care ethics committees, or health care situations that would have warranted involvement of an ethics committee. So, when I asked A and M what a health care ethics committee is and does, they both gave answers that leaned more towards business than health care. A believed that an ethics committee is comprised of lawyers and administrative executives who review and address issues or situations that might bring liability to the hospital. M also viewed the ethics committee as a guard against liability, but also thought the committee would include the hospital clergy. Both A and M thought the committee served more as an absolute dictator of action rather than as an advisor of action.

When I asked how an ethics committee would come to be involved in a situation, both A and M answered that a committee would get involved if a patient complained or if an employee was worried about knowing "the right thing to do" was in a controversial area. Both A and M used "pulling the plug" on life support as an example where an ethics committee might get involved. Interestingly, both A and M were as focused on the health system's liability and support for the health care workers' decision-making as they were about the patients' rights and protection. The focus on liability may be because both A and M have management roles within their respective organizations and were thinking more as managers than as potential patients.

Rosa Ruiz Rehabilitation Options

Case Overview

Rosa Ruiz is a Latina patient scheduled to be discharged to a rehabilitation facility for follow up treatment after surgery to repair a fractured hip. Mrs. Ruiz is a housewife whose husband and children are bilingual, but who, herself, only speaks limited English. Mrs. Ruiz's daughter, Adela, functions as the interpreter to facilitate communication between the medical staff and her mother. Currently, a social worker is trying to arrange post-operative care for Mrs. Ruiz. Mrs. Ruiz has expressed her preference to go to a rehabilitation facility that has other residents of Mexican ancestry, a staff that speaks Spanish, and is Catholic so she can go to Mass and receive communion. A review of Rosa Ruiz's case reveals ethical issues and implications not only for the patient, the patient's daughter, and the healthcare worker, but also for the healthcare system.

One of most obvious ethical challenges is presented by Mrs. Ruiz's limited ability to speak English. During her hospitalization, Mrs. Ruiz had to rely on her daughter, Adela, to function as an interpreter between herself and the medical team. Adela continued to function as an interpreter between her mother and the social worker when the social worker started working with Mrs. Ruiz on a discharge plan for rehabilitation following surgery, Adela continued to function as interpreter. Adela's role as interpreter presents a potential ethical issue because Adela can control what information is passed between her mother and the social worker without either of them being aware of the accuracy of the interpretation. Using family members to interpret for medical providers can also be an issue if the medical terminology is complicated and the family member simply lacks the knowledge and background to interpret accurately.

Respect for Autonomy

The social worker told Adela to inform Mrs. Ruiz that Our Lady of Guadalupe Skilled Nursing and Rehabilitation Center had a long waiting list for new residents and most likely would not be able to accommodate her within the required timeframe for her rehabilitation. Even though Adela knew her mother's "emphatically" stated desire, Adela chose to only translate some of what the social worker said and elected to omit information about the center. By omitting some of the information, Adela created an ethically compromised situation. Mrs. Ruiz effectively had her respect for autonomy violated by not having all the information she would need to make an informed decision about her treatment plan. Another ethical concern from the social worker's perspective is how to ensure a non-English speaking patient gets the correct information while remaining compliant with HIPAA laws. The social worker is responsible for ensuring maintenance of patient autonomy, but without speaking the patient's language or using a professional translator, the social worker is in jeopardy of unknowingly violating patient autonomy.

By allowing the use of a family member to translate for the social worker, the healthcare system put both the healthcare worker and the patient
in an untenable position. While the case does not indicate if Adela was
pressed into service because the health system lacked translators or if
Mrs. Ruiz simply felt more comfortable with a family member filling
that role, Adela's role as translator puts her into a position where her
autonomy is challenged. Adela is being forced into being simultaneously
both daughter and interpreter; roles where she will need to be neutral as
an interpreter, but empathetic and caring as a daughter. As mentioned
previously about using family members as interpreters, one does not even
know if Adela has the required medical terminology training to interpret
accurately. Adela should have the autonomy to decline acting as a translator without coercion or being forced into the role. Respect for autonomy
was, therefore, compromised for Adela as well as Mrs. Ruiz and the social
worker. Latino patients have differences in the way values are weighted
and how decisions are made.[01] Because the Latino patient has an identity
intertwined with the family and community, one must understand that
the typical concept of what constitutes patient autonomy must be rede-
fined for the Latino patient.[02]

Justice

Another ethical principle compromised in Mrs. Ruiz's case is justice. In
healthcare, we are normally concerned with distributive justice which, as
defined by Ozolins, is concerned with the distribution of social burdens,
as well as benefits and opportunities in a fair manner, so that one group

01 Peterson-Iyer, K. (2008). Culturally competent care for Latino patients. *Markkula Center
for Applied Ethics*. Retrieved from https://www.scu.edu/ethics/focus-areas/bioethics/resources/
culturally-competent-care/culturally-competent-care-for-latino-patients/
    02 Ibid.

in society does not bear the burdens of providing benefits while sharing in few of them, or receive more benefits than others in the community.[03]

Justice can also be conceived in terms of honoring a person's contextual reality which includes not only respecting a person's autonomy but also her family and cultural ties. In other words, rather than focusing on a person as an isolated individual, one should understand her contextual connectedness to other people and communities based on her cultural foundation.

Because of Mrs. Ruiz's cultural context and the paucity of facilities that satisfy it, Mrs. Ruiz is faced with compromised healthcare justice. One might consider Mrs. Ruiz's multiple, specific requirements for her preferred rehabilitation facility to be an excessively high requirement for just healthcare. However, one must concede that a patient should have ready access to healthcare within her cultural context that is equivalent in quality to that healthcare received by the cultural majority of the population. This is not the case with Mrs. Ruiz who seemingly has one option for treatment at a facility that matches her cultural context. Due to her lack of options, Mrs. Ruiz resigns herself in the end to just go home for care. The healthcare system and society as a whole would need to address this healthcare disparity through changes to healthcare policy.

The lack of resources for ethnic minorities would logically occur more often in smaller communities that have a limited amount of healthcare resources in general. Healthcare systems can institute cultural competency training for the staff, but language skills and cultural nuances would be outside the reasonable range and scope of such training. One solution might be to coordinate with a local or regional university that has a range of language and cultural studies programs. The healthcare system could

---

03 Ozolins, J. (2015). Ethical principlism. In J. Ozolins, & J. Grainger, (Eds.), *Foundations of Healthcare Ethics: Theory to Practice* (pp.33-50). Cambridge University Press. Kindle Edition, p. 46.

hire professors as consultants to provide translator and interpreter services for ethnic minority patients on an ad hoc basis either in person or
via video conferencing.

Companion Article

Fennell al 's work discussing Hispanics' access and quality of care in
nursing homes does little to address respect for autonomy among Latino
patients who require long-term care treatment. However, their discourse
does address the ethical concerns of distributive justice for Latino patients
in terms of nursing home use, racial and ethnic disparities in care access,
and current trends in the composition of nursing home residents.[04] Fennell et al. lay out the statistics behind the increase in utilization of nursing
homes by Latino patients and the closure of facilities by area with comments about implications for healthcare justice. While the authors touch
on the economics of long-term care and Medicaid reimbursement as a
root cause of the closures and a driver of the disparity in access, their only
recommendations for improving the justice disparity is "more resources"
and "policy proposals...that target at-risk nursing homes with multiple
innovative solutions."[05]

Conclusion

Mrs. Ruiz's case serves to highlight some potential ethical issues

---

04 Fennell, M.L., Clark, M., Feng, Z., Mor, V., Smith, D.B., & Tyler, D.A. (2012). Separate
and unequal access and quality of care in nursing homes: Transformation of the long term care
industry and implications of the research program for aging Hispanics. In: J.Angel, F. Torres-
Gil, & K. Markides, (Eds.), *Aging, Health, and Longevity in the Mexican-Origin Population.*
(pp. 207-225). Springer, Boston, MA.

05 Ibid, p 222.

inherent in providing healthcare to ethnic minorities. The issues are more involved and far reaching than a singular language or cultural problem and cannot be addressed with a simple, singular solution. The issues can spread out like fractures on a pane of glass, creating problems that require comprehensive, well-conceived solutions that account for the potential aspects of the situation. The easy answers are not always the best answers, as demonstrated by the use of family members as interpreters between medical teams and patient. Healthcare systems and communities need to come together and develop sufficient resources to serve the healthcare of the entire community including ethnic minorities. Through appropriate training, resource allocation, and policy development, society can minimize the potential for volatile ethical issues and maximize the just provision of healthcare.

References

Fennell, M.L., Clark, M., Feng, Z., Mor, V., Smith, D.B., & Tyler, D.A. (2012). Separate and unequal access and quality of care in nursing homes: Transformation of the long term care industry and implications of the research program for aging Hispanics. In: J.Angel, F. Torres-Gil, & K. Markides, (Eds.), Aging, Health, and Longevity in the Mexican-Origin Population. (pp. 207-225). Springer, Boston, MA.

Ozolins, J. (2015). Ethical principlism. In J. Ozolins, & J. Grainger, (Eds.), Foundations of Healthcare Ethics: Theory to Practice (pp.33-50). Cambridge University Press. Kindle Edition.

Peterson-Iyer, K. (2008). Culturally competent care for Latino patients. Markkula Center for Applied Ethics. Retrieved from https://www.scu.edu/ethics/focus-areas/bioethics/resources/culturally-competent-care/culturally-competent-care-for-latino-patients/

Case Study

For this case, you are a cardiologist and your patient is Sam, a fifty-eight-year-old man with known coronary artery disease and a long history of angina. Sam has come for his regular check up and complains of recent chest pain which has been typical during Sam's office visits over the last few years. Each episode was brought on by physical exertion and has been relieved with rest and a sublingual nitroglycerin tablet. You have performed stress tests and cardiac catheterizations in the past that have shown the presence of stable angina without major blockages or areas of ischemia. On this visit, your evaluation determines that Sam was having his typical angina with no need to change his medications or repeat invasive cardiac catheterization.

Normally, this would be the end of the appointment, however you recall the story about one of your fellow cardiologists who, in a similar clinical situation, sent a patient home without a cardiac catheterization. That patient died shortly thereafter of a heart attack, and the patient's family attempted to sue the physician for malpractice. Your judgment tells you that additional testing is not necessary, but now you have concerns about that holding up in court. Some cardiologists would agree with your assessment, but others would order a catheterization to protect themselves from potential litigation. You are also worried about the risk normally inherent with an invasive procedure as well as the financial impact for Sam.

Ethical Questions to Ponder

(1) When is defensive medicine a defensible alternative?

(2) How do the patients and/or the patient's family play into increasing the practice of defensive medicine?

(3) How do we balance the benefit and risk to the physician with the benefit and risk to the patient?

(4) If you decide to order the cardiac catheterization, how do you explain the reasoning behind the testing in light of informed consent?

(5) If you are inaccurately delineating the benefit of the procedure, then is the patient's consent actually valid?

Chapter 8

End-of-life Care
To Die, Not to Die & How to Die

End-of-life decisions have become increasingly complicated because as the potential for modern medicine to extend people's lives has increased and been generally well-received, these advances have also evoked ever more ethical quandaries. Not uncommonly, some patients have begun to decline the available life-extending interventions or even request euthanasia. Medicine, health care, and society seem to be unable to balance quantity of life gained with quality of life considerations. Moreover, the expenses of end-of-life care are very high and continue to rise.

Discussion Topics

What do you fear yourself about death and dying?

One of the aspects of death that can cause the greatest fear and anxiety is the state of non-existence. Even people with exposure to religion and a philosophical belief in an afterlife might be hard-pressed to maintain that belief when confronted by the end of physical life. Faith and hope can be strong motivators in life. However, having no hope for continuation of one's current existence and needing to rely on faith that there is another life right around the corner, whether that is eternal life of the soul or continual reincarnation until enlightenment, can be a hard pill to swallow. Fear is almost inevitable unless one's faith is absolute.

Another reason for fear of death can be attributed to the fear of missing out. One of the fears that I had when I was diagnosed and treated for ovarian cancer was the fear of missing my son growing up and experiencing all of the love and joy that I have as a parent. Another fear as a parent was the fear that I would not be around to protect, nurture, and provide for my son. I was also anxious about the sadness that my son would have at such a young age if I were to die.

There are a great many sources of fear surrounding death that go beyond the actual fear of the process of dying. People may fear the pain and sickness and trauma of death, but having personally gone through that, I think the fear of missing all of the wonderful things that life has to offer as well as the fear (guilt?) of causing pain and sorrow to one's family are some of the greatest fears I have regarding death.

Letting Go. Why is it so difficult for many health care professionals to "let go" of a patient? What are your personal experiences and expectations regarding this challenge?

Healthcare professionals can have a difficult time letting go of a patient at the end-of-life for a few reasons; some of these reasons are patient-based or influenced and others are physician-based or influenced. Physicians can be influenced by the circumstances of the patient's case and the context of the patient's life. For instance, a patient who is full of hope and optimism might cause the physician to buy into the "glass is half full" side of the prognosis and develop unrealistic expectations of his or her ability to pull the patient back from death. Also, physicians can be influenced by not wanting to crush a patient's expectations. This stems in part from the shift in patient-physician dynamics away from the traditional paternalistic mentality where the physician had complete control, to the current ideology where the patient plays a much larger role in directing her own care. The patient-centric expectation can influence the physician, similar to the way the "customer is always right" in the retail world.

I think the qualifier in the question that suggests we can focus our response on a specific population of dying patients points to an important factor in the reluctance of letting go. Professionally, I have been in certain practice settings where there was a stronger urge or push to not let go. In my current private practice as a cardiologist, the majority of my patients are older and have had chronic conditions that we have been treating for many years. Because the progression of the disease is slow and might not be the ultimate cause of death, the patient, the patient's family, and myself all have a certain comfort or level of understanding about the inevitability of death. However, during my cardiology fellowship, I practiced at a cardiac transplant center where the patient population was, demographically, wide-ranging. Many of the patients were struck with a cardiac disease unexpectedly in the prime of their lives and had many unrealized hopes and dreams. Several were young parents with small children. These patients and their situations had a strong emotional gravity that pulled on my heart and made me hang on longer, sometimes desperately, with a great deal of resistance to letting go.

I believe that this would carry over to other patient populations and disease states. If the patient and the physician have had time to come to terms with the death and the patient's life and family situation is not emotionally distressing, then the reluctance to let go might be mitigated. However, if the emotions are running high, then the physician can get caught up in that and have trouble letting go.

"Waiting. How does waiting relate to dying?"

The passive state of waiting described by Vanstone means that uncomfortable condition of being made receptive or subject to forces we cannot control such as illness, unemployment, workplace systems, and old age. One might think that the change of state from active doer to inactive receiver would not only represent a loss of physical independence, but also a psychological loss of value and self-esteem. However, the former state does not necessarily result in the latter state. As Vanstone states, "from the Christian viewpoint, it is never a degraded condition, a condition of diminished human dignity."[01]

Vanstone goes into great depth discussing Christ's shift from active to passive status as told in the Gospels of Mark and John. Even during that period when Christ moved "from the role of subject to that of object and from working in freedom to waiting upon what others decided and receiving what others did," He never lost His dignity or value. We see the ultimate value of Christ when we witness the thief on the cross asking

---

01 Vanstone, W. H. (2006). The Stature of Waiting. Church Publishing Inc. Kindle Edition.

Christ to remember him when He enters His kingdom (Luke 23:42).[02]

Vanstone notes that "a person who becomes a patient enters into passion; he becomes one who is done to, is treated: he becomes the object of the decisions and care and treatment of others."[03] Should our value in waiting for death result in lesser value? I would hope not. This is a troubling thought to consider given the state of healthcare across the US. We have seen an increased focus on production and cost containment over the last couple of decades, that puts a great deal of pressure on the healthcare team. It is not uncommon to hear an administrator say, "is the patient in room ####, bed # ready to be discharged yet? We really need that bed. So, if she/he is close let's get him/her out of here." This environment makes it hard to deemphasize the business side of medicine and focus on the human side of medicine.

If we have patients who are waiting to die and going through the stages of acceptance described by Copp, we need to be able to acknowledge that those stages are not absolutely defined and patients go through those stages at differing rates. How do we help our patients not only endure the waiting or passion before death, but also, hopefully get them to find peace and comfort for the majority of the time they are waiting. The waiting can be frustrating because of the feeling of powerlessness, but if we help the patient control as much of their lives and remove as many barriers as possible, then we might be able to maximize the patient's self-esteem and value during their passion.

'Doing to' versus 'being with'. As we have discussed earlier in this course, the primary mode by which health care professionals approach death and dying is through actions, rescue and even combat-like interventions. These engagements certainly can be

---

02 *The Holy Bible*, New International Version. Grand Rapids, MI: 2015.

03 Vanstone, W. H. (2006). The Stature of Waiting. Church Publishing Inc. Kindle Edition.

effective. But their value is limited by the inevitable mortality of human beings. How can health care providers sustain a relationship with dying patients without doing things to them?

The difference between 'being with' versus 'doing to' is related to both the intent of the person doing or being and the desires of the person receiving the doing or being. What is crucial is listening to and hearing the patient; understanding the emotions behind the needs the patient is trying to communicate. Otherwise, we are faced with a situation where the patient's desires are not recognized and the healthcare provider simply executes a treatment plan that addresses the physical needs as defined by the disease state. In that case, our actions as healthcare providers would be 'doing to' the patient rather than 'being with' the patient.

The same can be said when we take action that the patient does not want to receive. If a surgeon amputates a person's leg because of trauma or infection to save the person's life, then the patient will be grateful and the surgeon will have met the patient's desire. However, if someone is careless with a chainsaw and amputates a person's leg, then the amputee will say "look what you have done to me!" The desires of the person receiving the action or treatment are crucial to determining whether the action is 'being with' or 'doing to'.

Fostering hope might not be the most obvious aspect of caring for someone with a terminal illness. Hope can be considered fundamental to a life worth living and can change as circumstances change. One hope, such as hope for a cure, may become unattainable but may be replaced by another, such as hope to experience moments of connectedness with loved ones. By providing clear and honest communication and a listening, supportive ear, healthcare providers can help patients maintain hope. The key is to have the skill to foster and nurture hope that the final few months of life can be rich and fulfilling on an emotional and spiritual level.

In dealing with spiritual and emotional matters, quality care must be individualized, based on the patient's desires rather than being shaped by what the healthcare provider believes the patient ought to want or feel. There really is no single rule that can be applied to providing spiritual and emotional care for patients with a terminal illness. People vary widely in how they approach dying and how they choose to interact with their healthcare providers about the end-of-life journey. The basic requirements to being with the patient instead of doing to the patient, regardless of the patient's approach to dying, is for the healthcare provider to have an empathetic ear to hear the gravity of the patient's words, a caring heart so that what the healthcare provider hears matters, and the communication skills to encourage her to express herself and reassure the patient that she is being heard.

As I noted previously, intent is an important component of being with a patient. When the healthcare provider intends to meet not only the physical needs of a patient based on clinical guidelines, but also to meet the emotional and spiritual needs of the patient based on the patient's desires, then the healthcare provider has made significant strides toward 'being with' the patient rather than 'doing to' the patient.

References

Copp, G. (1998). A review of current theories of death and dying. Journal of Advanced Nursing, 28(2), 382-390.

The Holy Bible, New International Version. Grand Rapids, MI: 2015.

Vanstone, W. H. (2006). The Stature of Waiting. Church Publishing Inc. Kindle Edition.

Essay 13

SACRAMENT OF ANOINTING THE SICK: ARE THERE ALTERNATIVES TO SAVE MEDICAL ETHICS?

Introduction

Injustices in healthcare, as Dr. Martin Luther King, Jr. stated in a speech on human rights in 1966, is "the most shocking and inhumane... of all forms of inequality". In order to evaluate those injustices, one needs to employ "a moral lens—that can better discern the value-laden questions" that arise in the field of bioethics.[04] That moral lens is the coordination of the various theories of justice that create a mental and philosophical mindset to evaluate situations in one's environment. M. Therese Lysaught theorizes that the Sacrament of Anointing the Sick presents a polity that "enables us to think differently about who we are and what it means to flourish."[05] Lysaught argues that this polity based on the sacrament can illuminate "how deeply subject the sick are to the power of others and how the power exercised through medicine can be deployed either toward the ends of the world...or the toward the ends of the kingdom of God."[06] Lysaught contends that only through the

---

04 Rubin, D. (2010). A Role for Moral Vision in Public Health. *Hastings Center Report, 40*(6), p. 21.

05 Lysaught, T.M. (2006). Vulnerability within the body of Christ. Anointing the sick and theological anthropology. In C.R. Taylor & R. Dell'Oro (Eds.), Health and human flourishing. Religion, medicine and moral anthropology (Chapter 9; pp. 159-181). Washington, DC: Georgetown University Press., p. 176.

06 Ibid.

Sacrament of Anointing the Sick can the community be healed and "the sick in their woundedness are no longer seen as alien threats but rather rightly seen as gifts."[07] This paper will discuss the aspects of Lysaught's theory on the Sacrament of Anointing the Sick and argue that there are other Christian and secular alternatives available within healthcare to pull back medicine in the same way Lysaught believes the Sacrament of Anointing the Sick can.

Biblical basis of healing

The basis of healing as a Christian principle is well-established in the Gospels as it was the most important act performed by Jesus aside from the Passion. Jesus sent out disciples to precede Him in places He would be going with the instruction to be aware of conflict that lurks, travel discretely, greet each household with "peace to this household," and heal the sick.[08] According to the Gospel of John, the authorities used Jesus's acts of healing as one of the primary reasons to persecute and kill Him. Lysaught notes that Jesus responds by claiming that His healing acts are the core of the social order that is the kingdom of God and that healing is deeply entwined with the presence, proclamation, and politics of the kingdom of God.[09] Healing is a central part of the commission Jesus gives to those he sends out into the world to preach the good news of the kingdom and to embody it wherever they go.[10] One can say that healing, as seen by Lysaught, prepares the way for Jesus and is inextricably linked to peace, proclamation, and embodiment of

---

07 Ibid.

08 Ibid.

09 Ibid.

10 Ibid.

the kingdom.[11]

The Sacrament of Anointing the Sick

Lysaught argues that the Sacrament of Anointing the Sick is fundamental to the theological politics of medicine and making God's work real in the world. Lysaught argues "that a theological politics of medicine is found in the sacramental practice of anointing of the sick."[12] Lysaught further contends that "within the practice of anointing we find a radically theological hermeneutic—a theologically robust vision for interpreting medicine that, if enacted, can powerfully make real God's work in the world."[13] The role of sacramental worship which includes the Eucharist is central to the renewal of the Body of Christ in the world and in the spirit. As Lysaught notes, the practice of anointing is an indispensible starting point for meditating on anthropology and bioethics, as well as the application of theology to medicine and bioethics.[14] According to Lysaught, anointing has been elevated to the status of a Sacrament within the Catholic Church and stands as the church's primary response to illness and the attendant vulnerabilities.

Friendship with the World vs Friendship with God

Lysaught argues that friendship with the world is inferior to friendship

---

11 Ibid.

12 Lysaught, T.M. (2009). Medicine as friendship with God: Anointing the sick as a theological hermeneutic. Journal of the Society of Christian Ethics, 29,1: 173.

13 Ibid.

14 Lysaught, T.M. (2006). Vulnerability within the body of Christ. Anointing the sick and theological anthropology. In C.R. Taylor & R. Dell'Oro (Eds.), Health and human flourishing. Religion, medicine and moral anthropology (Chapter 9; pp. 159-181). Washington, DC: Georgetown University Press.

with God and only though friendship with God will medicine be practiced ethically. Lysaught notes that the Biblical foundation in the Gospels of the idea that "this fundamental polarity—between 'friendship with the world,' which is enmity with God and 'friendship with God'—is the central principle that organizes and shapes James' message from start to finish."[15] Once again Lysaught returns to the healing ministry of Christ as the basis for her argument that theology is the wellspring of ethics in healthcare. Lysaught continues by saying that to be 'friends of the world,' then, is to share this worldview, to see reality in these terms. It is to believe that the world is a closed system, a universe of limited resources, and it is to live as if this were true: competition, in rivalry, in maximizing one's share of scarce resources, even if my accumulation means that others go without, even if it means, because of this, their death. To be a friend of God, then, is to know and celebrate the fundamental character of reality, to proclaim this marvelous truth—that God exists, that God is true, and that consequently, the fundamental context of existence is gift—open, abundant, for-the-other not against-the-other.[16]

This would imply that secularists would practice medicine by prioritizing the physician's own wellbeing above the patient's wellbeing and through a contentious relationship rather than as a unified team fighting for the patient's best outcome. Lysaught goes on to claim that friendship with the world and with God are "mutually exclusive" and to "be a friend of God is to reject the world's way of construing reality and to reject the violence that it necessarily entails, [but rather] to be a person whose essential nature, whose entire character is oriented

---

15 Lysaught, T.M. (2009). Medicine as friendship with God: Anointing the sick as a theological hermeneutic. Journal of the Society of Christian Ethics, 29,1: 174.

16 Ibid, p. 175.

toward giving, not only to those who ask but simply 'to all'."[17] Once again Lysaught advances the claim that only through friendship with God and, by association, the Sacrament of Anointing the Sick is one able to give freely to one's patients.

Paul Farmer and Partners In Health (PIH)

Lysaught uses Paul Farmer and PIH to exemplify her point that the Sacrament of Anointing the Sick is central to instilling bioethics in healthcare through theological discourse. Paul Farmer is a physician and a professor of both medicine and medical anthropology at Harvard Medical School, the institution from which he concurrently earned in 1990 both his MD and PhD.[18] Farmer spends most of his time in Haiti where he serves the medical needs of the poor through his organization Partners in Health. However, in Lysaught's mind, Farmer is the example of a physician who is unqualified because he is not Catholic clergy and therefore unable to perform the Sacrament of Anointing the Sick. Interestingly, in Lysaught's words, "PIH strives to intentionally and concretely practice medicine within the framework of the Gospels."[19] By referencing the Gospels, which Lysaught holds as the wellspring of the healing ministry of Christ and therefore the Sacrament of Anointing the Sick, Lysaught acknowledges that one can aspire to the same all-giving Christ-like ministry without being ordained in the Catholic faith.

Lysaught goes on to commend PIH for their enduring efforts: "to counter the structural violence in which the poor are enmeshed is

---

17 Ibid.

18 Lysaught, T.M. (2009). Medicine as friendship with God: Anointing the sick as a theological hermeneutic. Journal of the Society of Christian Ethics, 29, 1: 173.

19 Ibid, p. 181.

to offer a peaceable space of healing and solidarity that can act as an antidote to the insidious effects of oppression."[20] Interestingly, Lysaught wonders what Farmer would think about her "claim that he and PIH embody a theological hermeneutic of friendship with God rooted in the sacramental practice of anointing of the sick."[21] Simply by making such a query Lysaught brings into question her theory that the Sacrament of Anointing the Sick is the only means by which medicine can hope to pull itself back from "friendship with the world" and the resultant violence. Lysaught confirms that "PIH is not a ministry of the church; it is not an ecclesial community; it is not in any obvious way sustained through Christian sacramental practices."[22] However, because Farmer uses religion as the basis for his practice, but not truly the Sacrament of Anointing the Sick, one can infer that the Christian belief in the healing of Christ can serve to bring about ethical behaviors in medicine rather than the strict application of the Sacrament of Anointing the Sick.

Secular vs Religious Basis for Medical Ethics

If one is to believe Lysaught, the sole hope for saving medicine from friendship with the world is the Catholic Sacraments, particularly the Sacrament of Anointing the Sick. As noted previously, the basic Christian belief in the Gospel of healing and the belief that we should love one another as God loves us can suffice to pull medicine back from the world's baser effects. One can also turn to the Jewish, Muslim, Hindu, and Buddhist religions, among others, to find traditions of caring for and healing the sick. In fact, many of the world's religious traditions place

---

20 Ibid, p. 186.

21 Ibid.

22 Ibid.

as much emphasis on the spiritual healing as the physical healing. "In the Hindu tradition, 'health' means the continued maintenance of the best possible working of the human body under normal, and sometimes even abnormal, environmental conditions. Hindu religious teaching on healthy living and ethical considerations culminate in spiritual objectives if the injunctions contained in the system are followed."[23] Buddhism is widely respected for espousing the virtues of benevolence and compassion and for its scruples for all living beings.

These religions have a respect for the human condition—both living and after death. This is similar to the Catholic idea of the Sacrament of Anointing the Sick and the Last Rites to prepare the soul at the end of life. While some religions believe in reincarnation, there still exists the idea that people have souls that carry on after death. The desire to protect the wellbeing of the individual as a vital part of the community is another common thread that streams through religious ideology. Eventually, those ideals filter down through all aspects of life among the religious adherents which would include the practice of medicine.

Even among socialist societies that have historically been atheistic in ideology, there is a society-wide need to provide medical care for each member of the society regardless of the nature of the illness or the standing of the person in the society. Humans seem to have an innate need to stop other members of their society from suffering whenever possible. The benefits derived from the Sacrament of Anointing the Sick can be achieved through the application of other bioethical principles and philosophies in the absence of religion.

If one were to review the values espoused by various medical associations such as the American Medical Association (AMA), one

---

23 Naidoo, T. (1989). Health and health care—a Hindu perspective. *Medicine and Law*, 7(6):643-647. Retrieved from https://www.ncbi.nlm.nih.gov/pubmed/2495404

would find that the principles would be in line with those principles found by Lysaught to be lacking in the world. The AMA puts forth principles as standards of conduct which define the essentials of honorable behavior for the physician. This includes among other principles, that a physician shall be dedicated to providing competent medical service with compassion and respect for human dignity, and that a physician shall recognize a responsibility to participate in activities contributing to an improved community.

Conclusion

So, it is not truly the Sacrament of Anointing the Sick that brings about ethical behaviors in medicine, but rather the basic tenets of Christianity that make the difference. If that is the case, then any ideology or source of morality, self-sacrific, and caring for the disenfranchised will also function as a wellspring for medical ethics. Again, if one were to view medical ethics through a moral lens, whether one employs a theory based on Rawlsian ethics or Kantian ethics, distributive justice or structural justice, cultural competence or cultural consciousness, etc., the simple act of considering the theories of justice causes one to assess and consider one's position and alter one's behavior accordingly. Once the process of evaluating ethical situations begins, one will be inclined to continue to consider various theories of justice when confronted with caring for the sick. Therefore, one can readily see that the Sacrament of Anointing the Sick is not the sole means for medicine to pull back from "friendship with the world" and the incumbent structural violence that would result. Rather, any Christian foundation or any secular ideology that emphasizes the welfare of the patient above the medical provider or the healthcare system will suffice to have an effect similar to the Catholic Sacraments.

References

Lysaught, T.M. (2006). Vulnerability within the body of Christ. Anointing the sick and theological anthropology. In C.R. Taylor & R. Dell'Oro (Eds.), Health and human flourishing. Religion, medicine and moral anthropology (Chapter 9; pp. 159-181). Washington, DC: Georgetown University Press.

Lysaught, T.M. (2009). Medicine as friendship with God: Anointing the sick as a theological hermeneutic. Journal of the Society of Christian Ethics, 29,1: 171-191.

Naidoo, T. (1989). Health and health care--a Hindu perspective. Medicine and Law, 7(6):643-647. Retrieved from https://www.ncbi.nlm.nih.gov/pubmed/2495404

Riddick, F. A. (2003). The Code of Medical Ethics of the American Medical Association. The Ochsner Journal, 5(2), 6–10.

Rubin, D. (2010). A Role for Moral Vision in Public Health. Hastings Center Report, 40(6):20-22.

Case Study

For this case, you are a neurologist and Fred is a patient of yours with amyotrophic lateral sclerosis (ALS) whom you have been treating for four years. Upon initial diagnosis, you explained that the disease progressed a little differently in each patient, but you had a frank discussion about the stages of the disease, what Fred could expect, and what would, eventually, cause death. Then you explained the type of interventions that could help manage Fred's illness, including physical therapy, speech and swallowing therapy, counseling, and medical intervention.

Fred, who lives alone, was able to maintain working as a computer programmer for the first couple of years after diagnosis, but eventually had to go on long-term disability. Fred continued to work with therapists and counselors as his condition deteriorated. Fred finally consulted a lawyer to plan for his end-of-life. Fred developed a living will stating that he does not want to be put on a ventilator or to receive a feeding tube when he was no longer able to swallow.

You see Fred in your office every few weeks. On the last visit Fred asked you to prescribe secobarbital and explain how to take the medication just in case his situation becomes unbearable because Fred wants to be able to commit suicide before he loses the ability to do it on his own.

Fred explains that he has no family and no one will try to coerce him to stay alive for the last few months, months which Fred is dreading. Fred goes on to say that he is not currently depressed or despondent, but wants to choose quality of life remaining over quantity of life remaining.

Fred goes so far as to suggest that you can write the secobarbital prescriptions over the next few months so that he can save up the medication and you will not be overtly liable. You feel torn because Fred's argument is sound, but as a physician you just cannot participate in helping him commit suicide.

Ethical Questions to Ponder

(1) Is it in the patient's interest to hasten death? Why?

(2) What role can we play in helping our patients clearly perceive and weigh their expectations and fears?

(3) Who can or should we turn to for support with patients' end-of-life questions and fears?

(4) How do we respect different religious or non-religious views on death and dying while still providing "appropriate" patient care?

(5) If we were to defer to the patient's individual interest, how might that deference create increased acceptability of PAS which will, in turn, cause harm to vulnerable populations?

Chapter 9

Home Healthcare:
Family, Friends, and Strangers

The appeal of home-based primary, acute, and palliative care has gained traction for its demonstrated potential to improve outcomes and reduce costs for our society's most vulnerable and frail patients. Administrators and policymakers must address the ethical dynamics endemic in the home health care environment for the patient, family, and providers.

Essay 14

Impact of Home Healthcare Environment on Patient Decision-making: Maintaining Balance among Bioethical Principles

Environment plays an integral role in a patient's decision-making process because resources and factors change as the environment changes. The dynamics of the home healthcare environment change the power structure among the patient, the patient's family, and healthcare providers, which affects patient decision-making. The root cause of changes in patient decision-making and patient treatment plans can be found in the difference between the home healthcare environment, as well as the institutional healthcare environment and the concomitant shifting of power from the provider to the patient and family. However, the family dynamics that shape and influence patient decision-making and the patient's autonomy can vary wide. This makes it difficult for the healthcare provider to develop or change patient care plans and to assess and respond to the patient in an ethical manner. The family social, cultural, and financial dynamics within the context of home healthcare will all need to be considered in this discussion of patient autonomy and decision-making. This paper will consider the ethics of a provider agreeing to changing a home healthcare patient's treatment plan to one that provides less healthcare benefit to the patient.

To focus the discussion on the family dynamics surrounding decision-making specifically related to ongoing, long-term homecare, the paper will be framed within the context of care for elderly, chronically ill, non-terminal patients who will receive care in their homes or the home of a family member. This is a reasonable group to consider because the patient will require constant, ongoing care with no foreseeable end to the situation, which can place greater strain on the family and force greater reconsideration of resource limits and changes to patient treatment plans. The patient's decision to request a change in treatment based on undue pressure exerted by the family instead of based on clinical soundness may result in decreased benefit to the patient. However, a patient may autonomously opt to pursue a course of treatment that is clinically less effective because the patient, without undue coercion, wants to spare her family from physical, financial, and/or emotional burden. One can consider a healthcare provider who complies with a patient's autonomous decision to elect a less efficacious treatment as ethical because respect for patient autonomy is maintained and, while health benefits may decrease, holistically, patient beneficence may be increased and the patient receives no direct harm, nor or is treated differently than anyone else in the exact same situation would be treated.

Home healthcare for children will not be considered in this discussion because the topic raises additional questions that cannot be fully addressed within the limits of this paper. The patient-family dynamics are quite different with a child patient than with an adult patient, and parents' legal responsibility for decision-making for minor patients would requires depth of analysis to which this paper could not do justice. Also, hospice patients will not be considered because end-of-life dynamics would confound the evaluation of long-term home care provided wholly or in part by the family and, again, warrants consideration that cannot be adequately addressed within the parameters of this paper.

Healthcare Provider Dilemma: Patient Under Pressure

During my medical ethics practicum with a home health care organization, we were presented with a case that exemplifies an ethical dilemma faced by healthcare providers in home healthcare. Our case was a white, 80-year-old male patient with Parkinson's Disease (PD) who, because he cannot manage self-care and the activities of daily living (ADL) on his own, moved in with his daughter so she could help care for him. During care assessment and treatment, the nurse noticed that the patient had developed a severe excoriation of his buttocks and scrotum. Upon inquiry, the patient reported that his daughter often failed to assist with the bathing and toileting which, according to the nursing staff at the practicum site, is not unusual for children taking care of parents. The patient was distraught by the situation, but did not want to do anything that would upset his daughter. Thus, he asked the nurse not to address the problem with his daughter. An important ethical question is whether the nurse should ignore the patient's request to not mention the problem—which the patient presumes would upset the daughter—and intervene with the daughter for the patient's welfare.

Patient Autonomy at Risk

The healthcare provider might face an ethical dilemma of providing care that was agreed to by the patient, but that results in less benefit to the patient when the provider knows that the patient has been unduly influenced or coerced by the family. Byrne, Goeree, Hiedemann, & Stern contend that it is vitally important to determine how a healthcare provider can identify the potential for negative impact on patient autonomy and decision-making secondary to that power shift from the patient to the family.[01] While the provider can attempt to advocate for the patient by intervening with the family and explaining why one treatment

---

01 Byrne, D., Goeree, M. S., Hiedemann, B., & Stern, S. (2009). Formal home health care, informal care, and family decision making. *International Economic Review, 50*(4), 1205-1242. doi:10.1111/j.1468-2354.2009.00566.x

is better for the patient than another, the final decision is with the patient and the provider can only give the care that the patient accepts. To maintain respect for patient autonomy, a healthcare provider cannot force a treatment on a patient that is counter to the patient's will. The patient may even decide that the effects on her family are more important to her than any possible consequences for herself and decide to sacrifice her interests for the sake of what she perceives to be the interests of her family. It would be appropriate to address these matters with her, but if she is clear that she wishes to make this sacrifice, that decision should be respected.[02]

A healthcare provider who accepts the patient's decision is displaying respect for patient autonomy because the provider is affirming the patient's "right to exercise their right to independently make choices and act according to their principles, values and beliefs, [emphasis added] without coercion from others."[03]

Sometimes there is only a small window of time to communicate with all the parties involved before a clinical care decision must be made. Freeman notes that "on the front lines of clinical decision-making, [physicians] do not have the philosopher's luxury of days or weeks for managing words. As a pragmatic doctor, [one is] forced to be a person of action or inaction. [One] must make a decision and advocate for the position [one] take[s]".[04]

Not every case, situation, or patient-family interaction can be

---

02 Smith, S., Pasquerella, L., & Ladd, R. E. (2008). Ethical Issues in Home Health Care. Springfield: Charles C Thomas, p. 11.

03 Ozolins, J. (2015). Ethical principlism. In J. Ozolins, & J. Grainger, (Eds.), *Foundations of Healthcare Ethics: Theory to Practice* (pp. 138 - 154). Cambridge University Press. Kindle Edition, p. 40.

04 Freeman, J. M. (2006). Ethical theory and medical ethics: a personal perspective. *Journal of Medical Ethics*, 32(10), 617–618. http://doi.org/10.1136/jme.2005.014837, p. 217.

antiseptically analyzed and managed. Time-constrained decisions may not follow any policy or procedure and one must be prepared to respond to those situations by relying on one's ethical base— virtue, deontological, or consequential - keeping in mind one's duties while remaining caring and compassionate and sensitive to "the nuances of each situation and to the family's cultural background and beliefs."[05] External circumstances, such as time constraints, can impact a patient's autonomy. If one views autonomy on a continuum, then one can consider a patient's decision, made within the context of the external constraints, at least partially autonomous if not fully autonomous.[06]

Variables that Affect Decision-making
Approaches to Analyzing the Variables

Several commentators on home healthcare and medical ethics point to the difference between home healthcare ethics and hospital system ethics as a useful tool for understanding issues confronted by home healthcare.[07, 08, 09, 10] Some of the aforementioned commentators, such as

05 Ibid, p. 218.

06 Ozolins, J. (2015). Ethical principlism. In J. Ozolins, & J. Grainger, (Eds.), *Foundations of Healthcare Ethics: Theory to Practice* (pp. 138 - 154). Cambridge University Press. Kindle Edition.

07 Byrne, D., Goeree, M. S., Hiedemann, B., & Stern, S. (2009). Formal home health care, informal care, and family decision making. *International Economic Review*, *50*(4), 1205-1242. doi:10.1111/j.1468-2354.2009.00566.x

08 Fry-Revere, S. (2008). The black sheep of clinical ethics: Home health ethics services. *Home Health Care Management & Practice*, *20*(4), 303-311. doi: 10.1177/1084822307310760

09 Hautsalo, K., Rantanen, A., & Astedt-Kurki, P. (2013). Family functioning, health and social support assessed by aged home care clients and their family members. *Journal of Clinical Nursing*, 22: 2953–2963. doi:10.1111/j.1365-2702.2012.04335.x

10 Smith, S., Pasquerella, L., & Ladd, R. E. (2008). Ethical Issues in Home Health Care. Springfield: Charles C Thomas.

Smith et al., take a more anecdotal, case-based review approach to the discussion of the home healthcare environment and how different factors impact patient care and treatment decisions. The anecdotal, experiential approach has some validity once sufficient data has been accumulated and root cause analysis has been performed. This approach is useful to indicate the changes in behavior and thinking that can occur when transferring to the home from an institution.

Others, such as Byrne et al., take a theoretical model, analytical data-driven approach to the discussion of elder home healthcare. Byrne et al.'s theoretical models based on data are an intriguing way to look at the decision-making process because one can get insight into the weight of different factors on the decision-making process. Byrne et al. reviewed models developed by other thinkers such as "Pezzin and Schone and Sloan et al. [who] present models that apply to families of any size, but only one child plays a role in the family's care decision."[11] Byrne et al. realized that in practice, more than one adult child in a family may participate in the family's care decision, and adult siblings may disagree regarding the best source of care for an elderly parent.[12] The potential disagreement among adult siblings and between adult children and elderly parents led Byrne et al. to develop a game-theoretic framework where the players include the patient, spouse, and all of the patient's children.[13] The game-theory model based on family dynamics sounds effective, but it does not take the home environment into account when modeling decision-making and behaviors.

---

11 Byrne, D., Goeree, M. S., Hiedemann, B., & Stern, S. (2009). Formal home health care, informal care, and family decision making. *International Economic Review*, *50*(4), 1205-1242. doi:10.1111/j.1468-2354.2009.00566.x

12 Ibid.

13 Ibid.

Site of Care—Home Versus Institution

In the home healthcare environment, long-term care treatment plans are influenced by social dynamics quite differently than in healthcare facilities. A shift in power dynamics occurs between patient and healthcare provider when patients' care moves from an institution to their homes. In the healthcare facility, the patient is expected to conform to the social structure, hierarchy, and rules of the facility which puts the medical team in the position of power and causes the patient to more often defer to the providers' recommendations about treatment.[14] The balance of power lies in the hands of the healthcare providers who bear the onus of ensuring that the patient receives just care that provides the greatest benefit from the treatment while showing respect for patient autonomy.[15]

As a physician, when I have given a patient treatment options, many patients respond, "I'll do whatever you think is best." One might question whether the "whatever you think is best" response is truly autonomous. If one considers autonomy to follow the three-condition theory, which states that autonomous action occurs when one acts intentionally, with understanding, and without controlling influences that determine one's actions, then if the patient understands the treatment options to the best of her ability and is not coerced into a specific treatment, one can consider the decision autonomous.[16] The deference to physician expertise in a medical office or a hospital can be the result of a mindset that recognizes where respect is due. But, if the patient-provider relationship

14 Fry-Revere, S. (2008). The black sheep of clinical ethics: Home health ethics services. *Home Health Care Management & Practice, 20*(4), 303-311. doi: 10.1177/1084822307310760

15 Ibid.

16 Ozolins, J. (2015). Ethical principlism. In J. Ozolins, & J. Grainger, (Eds.), *Foundations of Healthcare Ethics: Theory to Practice* (pp. 138 - 154). Cambridge University Press. Kindle Edition. Cambridge University Press. Kindle Edition.

is a true and well-functioning partnership, then there should be a give and take of both respect and deference between the two individuals. Respect and deference are indispensable in achieving beneficial and autonomous patient decisions.

The institutional healthcare environment can compromise a patient's decision-making ability due to the unfamiliar surroundings and the barrage of information coming from many healthcare providers. The chaos of the environment perceived by the patient can negatively affect a patient's ability to think clearly which decreases patient autonomy.[17] However, the institutional environment can also help to reinforce patient autonomy. Smith et al. describe a phenomenon associated with the institutional environment that a patient is insulated from the family's influence on decision-making and is more able to maintain autonomy.[18] Some have also noted that it is easier to maintain respect for patient autonomy in an institution because there are multiple other clinicians and staff members who can hold each other accountable and to whom the patient can appeal if she feels she is not being heard or if she feels she does not have a voice in her care. So, the healthcare team can intervene and overcome the lack of control the patient feels in an unfamiliar environment.

In contrast, a patient's home is an environment set and controlled by the patient according to her own lifestyle and cultural norms. The patient's perception of her ability to stand up for her autonomy and have some power in the clinical decision-making process tends to increase in

---

17 Fry-Revere, S. (2008). The black sheep of clinical ethics: Home health ethics services. *Home Health Care Management & Practice, 20*(4), 303-311. doi: 10.1177/1084822307310760

18 Smith, S., Pasquerella, L., & Ladd, R. E. (2008). Ethical Issues in Home Health Care. Springfield: Charles C Thomas.

the patient's home.[19] A patient's greater level of comfort in her home environment can lead to increased assertiveness and impact the clinicians' ability to implement care plans because of increased need to negotiate with the patient compared to the same care plan in a healthcare facility.[20] Even if the negotiation with the patient and the family is successful, the delay in implementation of treatment can negatively impact the health benefit derived by the patient.

Family Burden and Quality of Care

The literature also provides an extensive empirical review of many of the common ethical situations in the home health setting related to the family's involvement and the impact on patient care. Some papers delve into theories about causal explanations of how elder home healthcare is impacted by whether family members share common preferences, which family members participate in the decision-making process, which types of care arrangements are considered, and whether other decisions are determined jointly with parental care decisions.[21] Byrne et al.'s game-theoretic model for the provision of healthcare allows for both self-interest and altruism in the sense that family members weigh the value of their own effort and leisure as well as the health quality of the patient.[22] Byrne et al. found that while children care about the quality of health of their parent-patient, most children and children-in-law see

---

19 Fry-Revere, S. (2008). The black sheep of clinical ethics: Home health ethics services. *Home Health Care Management & Practice, 20*(4), 303-311. doi: 10.1177/1084822307310760

20 Smith, S., Pasquerella, L., & Ladd, R. E. (2008). Ethical Issues in Home Health Care. Springfield: Charles C Thomas.

21 Byrne, D., Goeree, M. S., Hiedemann, B., & Stern, S. (2009). Formal home health care, informal care, and family decision making. *International Economic Review, 50*(4), 1205-1242. doi:10.1111/j.1468-2354.2009.00566.x

22 Ibid.

the responsibility more as a burden themselves than a blessing to their parents.[23] The low tolerance of burden by the children results in "the tendency of spouses instead of adult children to provide care [because of] the lower burden experienced by spouses in the caregiving role instead of differences in care effectiveness between spouses and children or selfishness on the part of children."[24] These empirical findings are ethically relevant to the discussion because they provide insight into the intrafamily dynamics that can lead to coercion which influences patient decision-making and compromises patient autonomy.

Family members can be a vital aid to the success of a patient's home health treatment plan, but they can also present ethical issues and be a barrier that derails the treatment plan. In the latter case, family dynamics can differ dramatically depending upon whether the patient is staying in his own home or in the home of his children where the patient may feel like a guest and more of a burden.[25] Research by Byrne et al. indicates that the family's capacity to physically, emotionally, and financially provide care for their family member can influence the patient's decision-making.[26] Additionally, a family's communication skills can be tested during the home healthcare process and affect treatment plans and patient outcomes if not addressed early enough.[27] If the family is located at a distance from the patient, but still involved in the decision-making process, then communication can face some

---

23 Ibid.

24 Ibid, p. 1238.

25 Byrne, D., Goeree, M. S., Hiedemann, B., & Stern, S. (2009). Formal home health care, informal care, and family decision making. *International Economic Review*, 50(4), 1205-1242. doi:10.1111/j.1468-2354.2009.00566.x

26 Ibid.

27 Hautsalo, K., Rantanen, A., & Astedt-Kurki, P. (2013). Family functioning, health and social support assessed by aged home care clients and their family members. *Journal of Clinical Nursing*, 22: 2953–2963. doi:10.1111/j.1365-2702.2012.04335.x

hurdles that are hard to overcome.

I have experienced the scenario where distance and communication skills created barriers to care with a patient who had congestive heart failure (CHF) and required home healthcare. The patient had three adult daughters; one lived locally to the patient and two lived in other parts of the US. The two children who lived at a great distance from their mother, my patient - were both in the healthcare field: one was a nurse and the other was a pharmacist. The daughter who lived close to their mother was not in the healthcare field, but was responsible for providing daily care and tried to help communicate their mother's wishes both to me and to her sisters. The daughters who were in healthcare tended to not listen to the emotive desires of their sister and mother who had to deal with the situation not only in the day-to-day moments, but also with an eye to the endurance they had for the future. The dynamics among the sisters and their mother was contentious at times, causing their mother to frequently change her mind about what she wanted to do treatment-wise depending upon which daughter was the last to speak to her.

The confluence of the change in power dynamics among the patient, the healthcare provider and the patient's family can force each person involved in the situation to weigh ethical decisions about clinical courses of action and their role in the care. For example, the patient can suffer from decreased respect for autonomy by having her decision-making usurped by the family.[28] While people within a family will be naturally deferential to one another at various times during their lives based on the situation, there are occasions when a person defers because of undue pressure or because she feels vulnerable. Smith et al. note that a patient receiving home healthcare is more likely to defer to the family's

---

28 Smith, S., Pasquerella, L., & Ladd, R. E. (2008). Ethical Issues in Home Health Care. Springfield: Charles C Thomas.

desires against her better judgment or will out of fear of being overly burdensome or if the patient feels vulnerable in the home situation and does not want to "rock the boat". The patient can also suffer diminished health benefits if the healthcare provider does not notice that the patient is deferring to the family and not expressing her true wishes for her preferred, and possibly the best, medically-indicated treatment in favor of a treatment that is less medically indicated.[29]

Respect for Patient Autonomy Versus Family Member Autonomy

Respect for autonomy is not isolated to people who are patients. One can consider the patient's relatives who volunteer to provide care to the patient as acting first and foremost as members of that family. Because the relatives give priority to their roles as family caregivers, they will generally prioritize decision-making based on their status as a family member before their status as an individual. However, members of the family are also individuals who have a right to be treated with respect for their autonomy because of their status as a rational, sentient human being. If the duration of care or the intensity of care for the patient exceeds the amount the family member initially anticipated was willing to provide, then the family member might revisit the way he or she prioritizes patient versus self in the decision-making process. The autonomy of individual family members might be challenged at times by situations within the process of patient care due to pressure or coercion from the patient. While the patient is the central figure in the patient care plan, family members are not unaffected by the decisions being made. If the family members' individual autonomies are ignored, then they are simply and solely

29 Cho, E., Kim, E., & Lee, N. (2013). Effects of informal caregivers on function of older adults in home health care. *Western Journal of Nursing Research, 35*(1), 57—75. doi: 10.1177/0193945911402847

categorized as tools or implements for the realization of the patient's care plan. If one embraces the Kantian imperative of not using another person strictly as a means to another person's end, then one should understand that each individual family member should have his or her autonomy respected and each should enjoy the freedom to decide what he or she can and cannot do without coercion and guilt from the patient or healthcare provider.[30] This is not to say that family members cannot voluntarily make sacrifices for the patient's welfare. As long as those sacrifices are not coerced and the family decides what they are willing to do with full understanding, then they are not being used strictly as a means to an end, but they are acting as an autonomous individual joining in the care of their family. Ideally, the entire family, including the patient, will be in complete agreement about which treatment plan is the best for all involved in the home healthcare situation and will completely support the treatment plan selected.

Conclusion

While the treatment decisions made by each person or group involved in the treatment plan might differ based on the environment, a healthcare provider, regardless of practice environment, has the duty to maximize each of the bioethical principles of respect for patient autonomy, beneficence, non-maleficence, and justice. A healthcare provider can ethically provide a treatment that provides less benefit to the patient than an alternative treatment option if that treatment also maximizes respect for patient autonomy. For a patient to maximize autonomy in one setting, he might need to accept a lower level of healthcare benefit

---

30 Ozolins, J. (2015). Ethical principlism. In J. Ozolins, & J. Grainger, (Eds.), *Foundations of Healthcare Ethics: Theory to Practice* (pp. 138 - 154). Cambridge University Press. Kindle Edition. Cambridge University Press. Kindle Edition.

because the maximum potential level for each bioethical principle is dependent on the environmental factors present at the time the decision is made. This is reminiscent of the economic idea of the production possibility curve which depicts the maximum outputs for two products given a limited set of resources and inputs. In our healthcare example, the home environment supplied different resources and factors (i.e. family influence) than the institutional environment. Logic dictates that the maximum potential for the bioethical principles of respect for patient autonomy, beneficence, non-maleficence, and justice would differ based on the differences in resources and factors. Further analysis is warranted to determine ethical methods a healthcare provider can employ to mitigate deleterious factors endemic to the home healthcare environment that impact the decision-making process. It is said that knowing is half the battle, so knowing what factors affect the patient decision-making process and knowing how to address those factors will be a step toward increasing the maximum potential for all bioethical principles.

References

Byrne, D., Goeree, M. S., Hiedemann, B., & Stern, S. (2009). Formal home health care, informal care, and family decision making. International Economic Review, 50(4), 1205-1242. doi:10.1111/j.1468-2354.2009.00566.x

Cho, E., Kim, E., & Lee, N. (2013). Effects of informal caregivers on function of older adults in home health care. Western Journal of Nursing Research, 35(1), 57—75. doi: 10.1177/0193945911402847

Freeman, J. M. (2006). Ethical theory and medical ethics: a personal perspective. Journal of Medical Ethics, 32(10), 617–618. http://doi.org/10.1136/jme.2005.014837

Fry-Revere, S. (2008). The black sheep of clinical ethics: Home health ethics services. Home Health Care Management & Practice, 20(4), 303-311. doi: 10.1177/1084822307310760

Hautsalo, K., Rantanen, A., & Astedt-Kurki, P. (2013). Family functioning, health and social support assessed by aged home care clients and their family members. Journal of Clinical Nursing, 22: 2953–2963. doi:10.1111/j.1365-2702.2012.04335.x

Ozolins, J. (2015). Ethical principlism. In J. Ozolins, & J. Grainger, (Eds.), Foundations of Healthcare Ethics: Theory to Practice (pp. 138 - 154). Cambridge University Press. Kindle Edition. Cambridge University Press. Kindle Edition.

Smith, S., Pasquerella, L., & Ladd, R. E. (2008). Ethical Issues in Home Health Care.

Springfield: Charles C Thomas.

Case Study

Jane is an elderly woman with Parkinson's Disease who is being cared for by her son and daughter-in-law in their home. Jane's daughter-in-law is at home during evenings and over night, while her son works at night and is in the home during the day. Additionally, Jane has an aide who comes to the home five times a week for an hour or so to assist with bathing and dressing.

Jane is in your office today with her son and daughter-in-law for a routine appointment. You inquire of her son and daughter-in-law about any changes with ambulation or mental status. Jane's daughter-in-law comments that Jane is "doing okay, I guess, but she gets confused more easily now and we are worried about her balance when she gets up to walk."

Jane's son states that they are doing the best they can, but they are not sure what to do about Jane's wandering off as he found her wandering down the street a couple of times. Also, because he works at night, he sleeps during the day, and was once awakened by the smell when Jane tried to heat a piece of chicken wrapped in foil in the microwave.

You turn to the patient and comment that it sounds like she is being well cared for. Then you turn to the family and remind them per previous discussions that Jane's Parkinson's is fairly advanced and she will require more supervision and care as time goes on. You ask the family about their plans for around-the-clock care either in home or at a facility.

Jane's son becomes slightly tense and defensive as he repeats that they are doing the best they can for his mother, but they cannot afford to have 24-hour per day care. He also states that, "she took care of me, and now I'm taking care of her. We're never going to abandon her to some strangers!"

You respond by saying that part of your role in Jane's care is to inform her and her family about disease progression and future care needs which, you note, is only going to get more complicated and difficult. You acknowledge that prior to the progression of her dementia, Jane stated several times that she never wanted to go to a nursing home. However, with each visit, you are becoming increasingly concerned for Jane's safety.

Ethical Questions to Ponder

(1) With patients who suffer from cognitive decline, how can you best display respect by making them the center of the visit?

(2) To ensure patient autonomy by assessing the patient's capacity to make decision, how can you weigh the patient's cognitive ability with the nature of the decisions being made?

(3) What is the physician's role and responsibility to address caregiver burn out given that they are not your patients? How can you structure those discussions with the family?

(4) What are some of the benefits of approaching patients and family by having conversations with patients about activities of daily living instead of location of care (home vs. facility)?

(5) How can you best address safety concerns while differentiating between caregiver neglect and overwhelmed caregivers?

AFTERWORD

When I set out to compile the healthcare ethics topics and discussions for this book, I never would have imagined that we would have a front row seat to a pandemic the likes of which we have not seen since the Spanish Flu of 1918. The overwhelming significance of COVID-19 on our healthcare systems and our world prompted me to pause the publication of the book. As the pandemic took hold and shook the planet to its core, I started to see how this novel disease required novel responses from the healthcare system and society as a whole. Some of the impacts and issues we faced were fairly standard fare for healthcare ethics such as end of life care, rationing of scarce medical resources, and so forth. However, what truly intrigued me were some of the ethical dilemmas that are unique to a community enduring a long-term battle with a novel disease that has no epidemiologic history, no known treatment and no vaccine. We have literally been learning something new about COVID-19 every day for the last seven month (at the time of writing) which has required us to change our mitigation plans and courses of action each and every day. This has caused confusion, stress, and anxiety across our populace. All of these factors combine to warrant an examination of how COVID-19 has created unique situations for healthcare ethicists and what we need to consider as we work our way through this pandemic.

As I stated, the COVID-19 pandemic has presented the healthcare community with a novel situation with multiple shifts in healthcare decision-making and points of concern over the course of the last several months. Healthcare ethics has been confronted by this unusual and novel situation, requiring the development of different approaches to patient care that are both ethical and effective.

Initially, rationing concerns were focused on Personal Protective Equipment (PPE), ventilators, and potential treatments such as hydroxychloroquine, convalescent plasma, corticosteroids, monoclonal antibodies, and remdesivir which recently became the first FDA-approved treatment for COVID-19. The medical ethics surrounding the rationing of those items is quite similar to the rationing for organ transplantation. However, the need for rationing PPE, mechanical ventilators, and drug therapies is simplified because we can increase production of those items whereas the same is not true about organs for transplant.

A future rationing concern will be the distribution of COVID-19 vaccines once they become available, but the true current ethical dilemma regarding rationing of limited medical resources centers around the availability of ICU beds and the medical staff to care for the volume of patients. Early in course of the pandemic, much of the discussion focused on flattening the curve in order to preserve capacity within the healthcare system. Elective procedures were halted and routine patient visits were postponed. Unfortunately, as we enter the heart of the autumn season in the United States without a vaccine for COVID-19 to blunt the spread, we are experiencing a surge in coronavirus hospitalizations across the country with daily cases hitting all-time highs. The pandemic is putting new strain on local health systems, prompting plans for makeshift medical centers and new talk of rationing care to flatten the next curve of COVID-19 cases.

The healthcare community in El Paso, Texas has seen COVID-19 hospitalizations nearly quadruple to almost 800 in the last three weeks of October 2020, and their intensive care units reach full capacity. Exceeding the capacity of ICUs in a health system is a serious concern that has consequences many have overlooked. We cannot simply turn away COVID-19 patients who need ICU care settings for care. One solution to overcome the shortage of ICU beds during a pandemic is to quickly set up new ICUs. This requires available rooms in the hospital or the rapid construction of new units. We end up turning other areas of the hospital into temporary ICUs. Building new units has effectively increased the number of ICU beds by almost 100% in several countries and facilitated on-the-spot admission of large numbers of patients requiring mechanical ventilation. This was rendered possible by the dedication of volunteer health care workers agreeing to work in a new and singularly stressful environment. However, this option has been associated with a significant risk of reduced quality of care for several reasons associated with the difficulties in meeting nationwide standards for critical care facilities in this type of emergency context.

First, rooms converted from intermediate care units or post-operative recovery rooms are not adequately designed for the all the equipment and organization required in critical care. Second, healthcare professionals recruited to work in ICUs may not be adequately trained for specific and sophisticated ICU work despite the hastily improvised teaching sessions or "crash courses" organized to help them learn. Along with the risk of decreased skill level, insufficient training of these healthcare professionals increases the burden of work.[1] Third, in the context of a pandemic, highly sophisticated devices, especially ventilators, are frequently lacking even with the increased production we witnessed in the early stages of the pandemic. This leads to the use of inappropriate devices for the complex care of severe Acute Respiratory Distress Syndrome (ARDS) patients. Therefore, while the possibility of quickly setting up temporary ICUs permits the admission of large numbers of critically ill COVID-19 patients, there is a concomitant associated risk of downgraded quality levels of care and subsequent impaired prognosies, as shown in other situations.[2] Additionally, this type of organization may imply distributive inequality. The access to ICU facilities of heterogeneous efficiency might be handled as first come, first served, but in a practical sense could actually be first come, best served.

Another solution to the lack of ICU beds is transferring of ICU patients from inadequately equipped or undersized facilities in remote areas to available ICU beds in medical hubs. This is the standard process in New Mexico where COVID-19 patients in remote areas across the state are transferred to the University of New Mexico Health System in Albuquerque for care. To mitigate geographic inequalities, patient transfers from regions with dramatic shortages of ICU beds to areas less affected by the outbreak and with large numbers of available ICU beds and optimal material and ICU staff, have been implemented.

These long distance transfers require planes, helicopters or trains that have been specifically adapted to the care of critically ill patients. These patient transfers also necessitate the involvement of a large number of dedicated physicians and nurses to ensure the process goes smoothly and patient safety is maximized. This transfer strategy should be organized within a short period of time and should allow the transfer of a significant number of patients to increase the overall efficiency of the health systems involved. These transfers are associated with increased costs, but the failure of a health system due to a pandemic should not be the financial   responsibility of the patients or their relatives. The first ethical issue surrounding such transfers is related to the benefit/ risk balance. For the patient, the benefit of being in the hands of highly qualified teams is counterbalanced by the risk of clinical worsening during transfer. During patient selection, close attention should be paid to severity status: not too severe (transfer would be too risky), and not too well (to avoid unnecessary transfer). While informed patient consent should theoretically be part of the decision, in this case, in this case, most of the transferred patients were unconscious and unable to approve such a transfer, thereby ruling out the autonomy principle. Informed consent would have needed to be obtained from their next of kin. A second ethical issue concerns ICU departments accepting patients from a distant regions, thereby possibly increasing the risk of overburdening their own health system during an increased epidemic wave in their own area. If nothing else, the COVID-19 pandemic experience has shown that we did not have efficient predictive tools to precisely anticipate the kinetics of ICU bed requirements. Finally, such transfers may be associated with increased suffering and psychological trauma for the patients' relatives. Long distances and governmental limitations on travel during the pandemic will have negatively impacted, if not completely eliminated, relatives being able to be at patients' bedsides making communication about the patient's status impossible.

Healthcare professionals living through the COVID-19 pandemic are affected by distress similarly to the general population. Everyone is faced with the effects of lockdown and containment, the risk of illness personally and among family and friends, the lack of any discernable endpoint to the pandemic, and the lack of effective treatments specific to COVID-19. This knowledge void has forced healthcare professionals to constantly adapt to an ever-changing landscape of sometimes contradictory information which can result in feeling powerless and ineffective in their roles as healers. Mental and emotional stress is compounded by extended workloads, the overwhelmingly large numbers of patients, concerns about the suffering and potential poor outcomes of their patients, preoccupations about potential shortages of intensive care resources (including PPE), the fear of transmitting the disease to their loved ones, and apprehension about possible involvement in ethically difficult decision-making in resource allocation. This creates a perfect storm of extreme uncertainty and insecurity that has deleterious effects on the mental wellbeing of healthcare professionals.[3] Some studies have shown that frontline COVID-19 healthcare professionals have an increased incidence of psychological disorders compared with different control groups providing no direct care to patients.[4] In some countries, such as Italy or in France, for example, healthcare workers are applauded by the population each evening at 8 pm. Societal reward and glorification of the caring function appears to be a protective factor in the short term, however it may be dangerous for healthcare workers to fall into this trap: altruism has long since been recognized as a core value of this profession.

Insecurity and uncertainty are reflected not only on an individual level, but also on a collective level. The COVID-19 epidemic requires reinforcement of ICU teams with new staff members or even reorganization of units, weakening reference points and trust within teams. This context creates a feeling of vulnerability and loss of control for professionals.[5] Psychological support has been set up for caregivers, as many hospitals have initiated telephone hotlines, psychologists within units, relaxation sessions, meditation, discussion groups, and optimization techniques. These responses should ideally vary according to the phase of the pandemic.[6] Concrete measures to set up rest areas, to facilitate the logistics of meals, daily life, and the possibility of having leisure and relaxation time are optimally appropriate to the needs of caregivers during the crisis.

Throughout history, we have seen the detrimental impacts a pandemic can have on the mental health of affected populations. For example, research from communities affected by outbreaks of Ebola showed widespread panic and anxiety, depression resulting from the sudden deaths of friends, relatives, and colleagues, and survivor's guilt. As we journey through our collective COVID-19 experience, we have had to endure public restrictions and shutdowns, which are essential to halt transmission of the virus and stem the tide of COVID-19 infections.

However, these shutdowns have led to physical isolation, closure of schools, and widespread job losses. In addition, we cannot yet assess the impact that school closures will have had on the development and wellbeing of our children.

Across the country, irrespective of social or economic status, we have witnessed increased misuse of controlled substances and alcohol as people try to deal with the anxiety and depression caused by isolation. However, as with many other features of this pandemic, we find that not all people have been affected equally, when we examine the economic impact of COVID-19. People with salaried jobs are far less likely to be affected than those with informal, daily wage jobs, which include a substantial proportion of the workforce in areas of the country that rely on tourism and entertainment such as Central Florida. Also, frontline workers are experiencing increased workload and trauma, making them susceptible to stress, burnout, depression, and post-traumatic stress disorder.

Unfortunately, in late October 2020, we are seeing a significant increase in COVID-19 cases. Dr. Anthony Fauci, the director of the National Institute of Allergy and Infectious Diseases, believes that the US will not see any semblance of normalcy until the end of 2021 or even early 2022. As we approach winter in the US, we are averaging about 70,000 new cases per day compared to about 35,000 new cases per day in early September.[7] Moreover, eleven US states have reported their highest single day death rates since the COVID-19 pandemic began. With the availability of a COVID-19 vaccine still months away, there is a chance that a significant portion of US society will not be vaccinated until mid-2021.

Dr. Jonathan Renier, a professor of medicine at George Washington University, opines that the US may see 500,000 COVID-19 deaths if US citizens do not improve their execution of mitigation measures. Fauci echoed this sentiment saying, "If you don't want to shut down, at least do the fundamental, basic things, which are really the flagship of which is wearing a mask. We can't have this very inconsistent wearing that you see, where you see some states that absolutely refuse to wear a mask."

With much of the US experiencing COVID-19 fatigue, the nation is faced with an ethical dilemma of balancing policies, mandating fundamental mitigation measures and a nationwide shutdown. If the populace will not practice the fundamentals of wearing appropriately constructed masks properly, distancing from other people by six feet or more, avoiding crowds in congregate settings, spending more time doing outdoor activities, and frequent handwashing, then the government will need to consider a shutdown. So, what are the ethical implications of a national shutdown, which would increase mental health issues, in order to prevent the spread of a disease with only one approved treatment and no vaccine? We, as a collective society, have become so accustomed to minimal personal restrictions, that we forget our desire for autonomy cannot supersede our duty for nonmaleficence. As the ethical principle of nonmaleficence states, we have an obligation to not inflict harm on others.[8]

By now, we should know full well that our ability to work our way through the COVID-19 pandemic will require development of effective vaccines in addition to treatments and strict adherence to the mitigation measures as I mentioned previously. The achievement of effective COVID-19 vaccine research and development would bring an increase in the level of hope and encouragement, that we can truly cope with the COVID-19 pandemic. Two aspects of the research and development process that should be balanced are the immediate necessity for speed of vaccine research and the inherent need for protection of research subjects, the latter of which is the foremost concern of research ethics.

Normally, vaccine development takes years, even decades before a viable vaccine is on the market for widespread use. The trial process for vaccines consists of several steps which need to be conducted systematically and in a measurable stride. The length of this process is correlated with the nature of the vaccine itself, which is to protect healthy people from being infected by pathogens. Adverse events and deleterious effects will not be tolerated. Vaccines are not the same as drugs that are consumed by the sick; the risk–benefit analysis for prescription drugs and vaccine administration is different.

The value of a COVID-19 vaccine to the entire world is so high that President Donald Trump called for development of a plan to streamline the development and production of a vaccine. This resulted in the establishment of Operation Warp Speed (OWS) which is a collaborative effort among the US Department of Health and Human Services (HHS), the Department of Defense (DoD) and the private sector to accelerate the testing, supply, development, and distribution of safe and effective vaccines, therapeutics, and diagnostics to counter COVID-19 by January 2021. In order to accelerate the development of a vaccine, efforts must be focused on streamlining the entire process. Unfortunately, streamlining may have consequences for the traditional ethics of vaccine research and development, especially the core principles of beneficence and nonmaleficence.

The need to protect hundreds of millions of Americans has pushed the government and the public to an extremely high expectation for the new vaccine—both timing and access. The overriding expectation may influence the objective judgement typically required of candidate vaccine safety. Protecting lives should be the top priority.

Throughout the COVID-19 pandemic, all societies have seemed to expect a breakthrough in medical and health technology to stem the tide of the disease and the concomitant morbidity and mortality. In a situation where understanding of the new disease is poor and no satisfactory medical technology is available for prevention and treatment, we are naturally led to think that it is better to do something, anything than to do nothing. This is going to make judgements about safety among decision-makers in the development and production processes more prone to missteps and rash choices.

One of the crucial steps of vaccine development is the challenge test, which is used to measure the potential protection of the candidate.[9] With COVID-19, we will need to depart from the typical animal test model and go straight to human testing because the virus does not produce the same clinical course and outcomes across species. While the choice to start testing with humans might sound unsafe, we are confronted with a disease that has no true treatment as Remdesivir has recently received FDA approval, but data is limited; our options are extremely limited.

So, how can we do this experiment within the current ethical review process given the fact that other similarly developed vaccines (i.e. malaria, typhoid, cholera) were for diseases with proven treatments? Those test subjects who had adverse effects of the disease after the experiment could be "rescued" with the treatment if needed. That safety net does not exist with COVID-19 because, as noted, there are no standard treatments for it yet.

The safety, tolerability, and efficacy of the vaccines should be obtained from different geographic areas, ethnicities, prevalence and varieties of the virus circulating in those areas. We know that there are already multiple different genomes for the SARS-CoV-2 virus. The inclusion of vulnerable populations in the development of the vaccine should be reviewed in order to prevent exploitation, or even the perceived exploitation, of those populations.

Another concern is the availability of an adequate health facility and system to ensure that trial subjects their families, as well as communities have access to treatment and proper care in case of serious adverse events related to the trial outcomes. We will inevitably recruit vulnerable subjects into the vaccine trials, so instituting protective measures to safeguard them as well as marginalized, populations should be paramount to the review of trials. We must be cautious about excluding vulnerable groups under the misconception that we are protecting them because that may diminish trial validity due to selection bias. If we are going to exclude them, there needs to be reasonable scientific and ethical justification.[10]

It should go without saying, but subjects should have initial access to the developed vaccine following the conclusion of the trials and production. This is part of their direct advantage for their involvement in the research. Also, there are COVID-19 vaccine development trials across the globe with many trials involving multiple countries and intercontinental research in order to recruit test subjects from different countries and regions. Therefore, access to COVID-19 vaccines after the conclusion of a trial should be expanded beyond the country in which the trial is based to include the broader global population. In fact, access to the COVID-19 vaccine should have been addressed from the very beginning of research design. The truncated development pathway and limitations on test subjects due to the nature of the disease raises ethical issues that must be addressed by everyone engaged in the research, development, and production processes. The urgent need for an effective COVID-19 vaccine to save humankind must not supersede the need to ensure that research ethics are maintained.

Many ethical challenges have complicated the current COVID-19 pandemic. Politicians have injected their political interests into the way we have approached the pandemic on all levels of society which has created confusion and ineffective implementation of mitigation measures. The news media have sensationalized the statistics and the response to the government's decisions which has injected even more emotion into a healthcare emergency that requires an ethical, rational medical solution. Tangential to the mental health ethics involved with the impact of an economic shutdown are the political and business ethical decisions confronting society about how to reopen the economy and which economic needs will be prioritized. Post-pandemic medical needs for mental health care, for the backlog of less serious conditions now needing care, and for an exhausted and disheartened medical community will need attention. Even more than seven months into our journey through the COVID-19 pandemic in the US, the disease has evolved and remained largely unpredictable. The end of the pandemic and the long-term effects of both the disease and the collateral damage due to mitigation measures are still unknown. Healthcare ethicists and other healthcare professionals must take the lessons we have learned and those we will continue to learn from Covid-19 in the coming months or even possibly years and put them into practice as soon as possible to ensure that we are maintaining respect for autonomy, beneficence, nonmaleficence, and justice across our entire society. Only by learning from our experiences and implementing better, more ethical processes will we be better equipped to handle the next pandemic that comes our way.

References

1. Adams LM, Melius J. Prepared to respond? Exploring Personal disaster preparedness and nursing staff response to disasters. Disaster Med Public Health Prep. 2020;7:1–6.

2. ESICM Working Group on Quality Improvement, Valentin A, Ferdinande P. Recommendations on basic requirements for intensive care units: structural and organizational aspects. Intensive Care Med. 2011;37(10):1575–87.

3. Chen Q, Liang M, Li Y, Guo J, Fei D, Wang L, et al. Mental health care for medical staff in China during the COVID-19 outbreak. Lancet Psychiatry. 2020;7(4):e15–6.

4. Tan BYQ, Chew NWS, Lee GKH, Jing M, Goh Y, Yeo LLL, et al. Psychological impact of the COVID-19 pandemic on health care workers in singapore. Ann Intern Med. 2020. https://doi.org/10.7326/M20-1083.

5. McAlonan GM, Lee AM, Cheung V, Cheung C, Tsang KWT, Sham PC, et al. Immediate and sustained psychological impact of an emerging infectious disease outbreak on health care workers. Can J Psychiatry Rev Can Psychiatr. 2007;52(4):241–7.

6. Xiang Y-T, Yang Y, Li W, Zhang L, Zhang Q, Cheung T, et al. Timely mental health care for the 2019 novel coronavirus outbreak is urgently needed. Lancet Psychiatry. 2020;7(3):228–9.

7. Institute for Health Metrics and Evaluation, COVID-19 Projections; https://covid19.healthdata.org/united-states-of-america?view=total-deaths&tab=trend; (Accessed October 29, 2020).

8. Jahn W. T. (2011). The 4 basic ethical principles that apply to forensic activities are respect for autonomy, beneficence, nonmaleficence, and justice. Journal of chiropractic medicine, 10(3), 225–226. https://doi.org/10.1016/j.jcm.2011.08.004.

9. Wibawa, T. (2020), COVID-19 vaccine research and development: ethical issues. Trop Med Int Health. doi:10.1111/tmi.13503.

10. WHOd. Ethical standards for research during public health emergencies: Distilling existing guidance to support COVID-19 R&D. 2020. https://apps.who.int/iris/handle/10665/331507.